VISUAL &
VESTIBULAR
CONSEQUENCES OF
ACQUIRED BRAIN
INJURY

Editors
Irwin B. Suchoff, O.D., D.O.S.
Kenneth J. Ciuffreda, O.D., Ph.D.
Neera Kapoor, O.D., M.S.

OPTOMETRIC EXTENSION PROGRAM FOUNDATION, INC.

Copyright © 2001 Optometric Extension Program Foundation, Inc.

Printed in the United States

Published by the Optometric Extension Program
1921 E. Carnegie Ave., Suite 3-L
Santa Ana, CA 92705-5510

Library of Congress Cataloging-in-Publication Data
Visual & vestibular consequences of acquired brain injury / editors, Irwin B. Suchoff,
Kenneth J. Ciuffreda, Neera Kapoor
        p. ; cm.
    Includes bibliographical references and index.
    ISBN 0-943599-42-3 (alk. paper)
    1. Ocular manifestations of general diseases. 2. Vestibular apparatus--Diseases.
    3. Brain damage--Complications. I. Title: Visual & vestibular consequences of
    acquired brain injury. II. Suchoff, Irwin B. III. Ciuffreda Kenneth J., 1947-
    IV. Kapoor, Neera.
    [DNLM: 1. Brain injury--complications. 2. Optometry--methods. 3. Vestibular
    Diseases--etiology. 4. Vestibular Diseases--rehabilitation. 5. Vision
    Disorders--etiology. 6. Vision Disorders--rehabilitation. WL 354 V8347 2001]
    RE65 .V57 2001
    617.7'1--dc21

                                                    2001055181

Optometry is the health care profession specifically licensed by state law to prescribe lenses, optical devices and procedures to improve human vision. Optometry has advanced vision therapy as a unique treatment modality for the development and remediation of the visual process. Effective vision therapy requires extensive understanding of:

- the effects of lenses (including prisms, filters and occluders)
- the variety of responses to the changes produced by lenses
- the various physiological aspects of the visual process
- the pervasive nature of the visual process in human behavior

As a consequence, effective vision therapy requires the supervision, direction and active involvement of the optometrist.

Table of Contents

Foreword

No one expects to acquire a brain injury. No one awakes and consciously or subconsciously plans on such a negative life-altering experience. We typically decide to stay out of harm's way in our daily activities whether at school, work, home or sporting activities. Nevertheless, unforeseen tragedies can occur despite our best efforts. The most recent unsettling example is the September 11, 2001 terrorist activity in New York City, Washington, DC, and Somerset, Pennsylvania. We are acutely aware of the many lives that were lost. Another aspect of these tragic events has received much less attention: many lives may have been altered by insult to the brain from flying debris, not necessarily received at the immediate scene of the accident. Incidents of debris-caused head injury, blocks away from the accident, were reported.

Although the effects of an acquired brain injury (ABI) can be immediately evident, the behavioral consequences of some injuries may not surface for some time, creating far-reaching challenges for the victims and those professionals who attempt to determine the genesis of the changed behavior as well as how to resolve it. Less cataclysmic on a grand scale, but devastating nevertheless, are damages from car and motorcycle injuries, bicycle injuries, pedestrian accidents, work mishaps, sports injuries, fights, accidents that occur in the comfort of one's own home such as falls, or cerebrovascular accident (stroke) that can happen anywhere at any time.

When I lecture about ABI, I include my "One Second Theory." Quite simply stated, we are each one second away from being someone's patient. Our background or status in the environment does not preclude anyone from the premise of this theory. And in fact, in my work with patients who have incurred ABI, I have examined and treated individuals of all ages, from all walks of life, all levels of education, all economic strata, and sometimes those I have known socially and/or professionally. The constellations of symptoms are as diverse and complex as each patient.

Recently I took my three-year-old daughter to the local library story time where parents experience the joy of seeing their children listening to stories. I recognized one of the dads as a previous patient who had been referred to me because he had incurred a head trauma. I did not know him prior to the time he sought my care. He is a young man who was in good health when, as a helmeted bicycle rider, he was struck from behind by a car.

While intermittently watching him during this 45-minute library session, I observed that he was still suffering from the aftereffects of his injury; he appeared to have difficulty sitting and attending. Despite his obvious discomfort, he still showed the same affection for his daughters as I did for mine while we listened to the stories. Afterwards, I identified myself, and we had an opportunity to talk to each other not as doctor and patient, but dad to dad. He was doing better, but we both decided that he and I will still need to do some additional work. However, watching him with his daughters gave me a different perspective and a far better appreciation for the "One Second Theory."

The authors of this book have developed expertise in the rehabilitation of ABI patients and have far more experience in this regard than most of us who will have the privilege to read their chapters. Gathering this collective that represents professionals involved in the visual and vestibular rehabilitation of ABI patients under one cover is a feat all by itself. But to then coordinate their works in a cohesive manner makes the reading pleasurable. Further, because the material is presented in a manner that is reflective of current optometric involvement in this area of rehabilitation, the book is both informative and clinically relevant.

In the first two chapters, the reader is given an orientation to ABI from the optometric and medical perspectives. The rest of the book is composed of topics that are particularly relevant to the rehabilitation of the visual and vestibular consequences of ABI. Although there are many approaches to the evaluation and remediation of this population, the editors made a conscious effort to choose those topics that could easily be integrated by the reader. To those ends, case reports are presented, which can be used by the reader to begin to understand how this knowledge can be put into practical use. I would challenge the reader to utilize the knowledge gained in the chapters, as well as past experience, to determine a therapeutic regimen for these patients based on the history and clinical findings presented, comparing that to what actually occurred.

This work is not offered as a textbook. Rather, it presents a picture of the current state of optometric activities in the visual rehabilitation of ABI patients, which is a work in progress. The observant reader will notice a lack of total conformity that exists in this very challenging field. This is evidenced by differing statistics and terminology in some of the chapters. I submit that these differences are an indication of the complexity of the subject matter. For example, differing estimates of the incidence and prevalence of ABI are a product of differing criteria and statistical methods. And although the editors clearly state their concept of ABI, other authors of this book use a broader definition. These differences are not contradictory; they are indicative of the experiences and operational necessities that each rehabilitative profession brings to the team. As greater interprofessional communication develops in the clinical setting, from the lecture platform and in the literature, more uniformity will result.

Optometry should be proud of its past and continuing contributions to the ABI rehabilitation team. We understand the dynamics of all aspects of the visual process and how they affect the person's overall behavior and function. Integrating that information into the inter- and intra- professional team therapeutic plans and goals, has, I believe, contributed to an enhanced quality of life of many ABI patients. I further posit that this book will serve to promote greater understanding, both within and outside the profession, of the role optometrists can productively play in the rehabilitation of these patients. The charge to readers of all involved professions is to take this information and use it as a platform to enhance our models of rehabilitative care.

Paul B. Freeman, O.D.
Sewickley, Pennsylvania

Preface

This book is the outgrowth of a symposium conducted at the American Academy of Optometry's annual meeting in 1999. All who presented were asked to submit extended versions of their talks, first as journal articles, and later as chapters when it was determined that a book was more appropriate. Another individual, who had been invited to present at the meeting but could not attend, agreed to submit a chapter.

Thus, this book has its roots in optometry. However, the subject matter, for the symposium and the book, necessitated that other rehabilitation professionals be involved. This was done to accurately represent the interdisciplinary clinical nature and realities of optometric involvement in the care of patients with acquired brain injury (ABI). Although not every rehabilitative discipline has a chapter authored by one or more of its members, we feel that virtually all have been recognized in this book.

One goal of this work is to provide optometrists with a broad understanding of ABI, its ocular and visual consequences, the developing clinical strategies that address these consequences, and some of the current pertinent optometric research. This information is contained in the first 10 chapters. While this goal is primarily oriented toward optometry, we believe that it will be valuable for other professionals dedicated to the rehabilitation of patients who have incurred ABI. The majority of these chapters should alert these health care providers to the contributions optometrists make to improve the functional abilities and quality of life of these patients.

The final three chapters are included because of the developing role of optometrists in the rehabilitation of individuals who suffer from dysfunctions of the vestibular system. These dysfunctions are not infrequently sequelae of ABI. As those professionals who specialize in this area become more aware and sophisticated regarding the role that vision plays in the maintenance of spatial orientation and balance, they are increasingly calling on optometrists to become active members of the rehabilitation process. This is especially meaningful for optometrists who subscribe to the model of vision proposed by A. M. Skeffington, the founder of the Optometric Extension Program (OEP). In his paradigm, developed during the early part of the last century, vision is not conceptualized as an isolated entity: rather, it is the product, or emergent, of the interaction of several other physiological processes, the first being termed "anti-gravity."[1] There is clear evidence that Dr. Skeffington understood that this name was synonymous with the vestibular system.[2] Readers of these three chapters will have an enhanced appreciation and understanding of the anatomical, neurophysiological and clinical relevance of the interactions of the visual and vestibular systems in the interest of human spatial orientation and balance. This constitutes our second goal.

Finally, our most ambitious goal is to increase inter- and intra- professional knowledge of the evolving and unique role that optometrists fill in the rehabilitation of patients who have sustained ABI. We most particularly hope that this book will serve to attain that goal.

References
1. Skeffington AM. The totality of vision. Arch Am Acad Optom 1957; 34(5): 5.
2. Birnbaum MH. Optometric Management of Nearpoint Vision Disorders. Boston: Butterworth-Heinemann, 1993:34.

Irwin B. Suchoff, O.D., D.O.S.
Kennesaw, Georgia
Kenneth J. Ciuffreda, O.D., Ph.D.
Neera Kapoor, O.D., M.S.
New York City
September 2001

Contributors

Kenneth J. Ciuffreda, O.D., Ph.D.
Chair, Department of Vision Sciences and Distinguished Teaching Professor, State University of New York, State College of Optometry. Associate Member, Graduate Faculty in Biomedical Engineering, Rutgers University.

Allen H. Cohen, O.D., FAAO, FCOVD
Chief Optometry Service, Northport VA Medical Center
Professor of Clinical Optometry, State University of New York, State College of Optometry. Private Practice: Specializing in Vision Rehabilitation, Lake Ronkonkoma, NY.

Paul B. Freeman, O.D., FAAO, FCVOD, Diplomate, Low Vision
Chief, Low Vision Services, Allegheny General Hospital, Pittsburgh, PA, limited to the evaluation and management of visually impaired, brain-injured, and mutliply handicapped individuals. Consultant Health South Harmarville Rehabilitation Center, Harmar, PA, The Children's Institute of Pittsburgh, Pittsburgh, PA, Western Pennsylvania School for Blind Children, Pittsburgh, PA . Editor *Optometry, Journal of the American Optometric Association* (1999-present).

Michael Gallaway, O.D., FCOVD
Associate Professor at Pennsylvania College of Optometry, Private Practice: Specializing in Vision Therapy and Children's Vision, Cinnaminson, NJ.

Rosamond Gianutsos, Ph.D., FAAO, CDRS
Adjunct Associate Professor, State University of New York, State College of Optometry, Head Trauma Vision Rehabilitation Unit. Previously on the faculty of Adelphi University. Private Practice: Specializing in Cognitive Rehabilitation, Sunnyside, NY.

Wayne A. Gordon, Ph.D., ABPP
Professor of Rehabilitation Medicine, Mount Sinai School of Medicine, New York, NY. Dr. Gordon was formerly at Rusk Institute, New York University Medical Center.

Ying Han, M.D., Ph.D.
Research Associate, Department of Vision Sciences, State University of New York, State College of Optometry.

Lynn Fishman Hellerstein, O.D., FCOVD, FAAO
Adjunct Professor of Optometry, Illinois College of Optometry and Pacific University College of Optometry. Private Practice: Specializing in Vision Rehabilitation, Englewood, CO.

Mary R. Hibbard, Ph.D., ABPP
Associate Professor, Department of Rehabilitation Medicine, Mount Sinai School of Medicine. Dr. Hibbard was formerly at Rusk Institute, New York University Medical Center.

Mary M. Jackowski, Ph.D., O.D.
Research Associate Professor, Department of Ophthalmology and Department of Physical Medicine and Rehabilitation, State University of New York, Health Science Center, Syracuse. Adjunct Associate Professor, Department of Psychology, Syracuse University. Co-ordinator of Low Vision Services, Veterans Administration Medical Center, Syracuse, NY.

Neera Kapoor, O.D., M.S.
Assistant clinical professor of optometry and the director of the Raymond J. Greenwald Vision Rehabilitation Center at the State University of New York, State College of Optometry.

Barbara Kenner, Ph.D.
Adjunct Professor, Rehabilitation Psychology and Clinical Neuropsychology, Department of Rehabilitation Medicine, Mount Sinai School of Medicine, New York, NY. Private Practice: Neuropsychological Assessment and Consultation Service, New York, NY.

Stephen Leslie, B Optom, FACBO, FCOVD
National President of the Optometrists' Association of Australia 1991-1992. Currently National Vice President of the Australasian College of Behavioural Optometrists. Private Practice: Specializing in Vision Rehabilitation, Perth, Western Australia.

David Malamut, M.A., P.T.
Rusk Institute of Rehabilitation Medicine, New York University Medical Center.

Edwin F. Richter, III, M.D.
Associate Clinical Professor, Rusk Institute of Rehabilitation Medicine, New York University Medical Center.

Steven A. Rosen, M.D.
Director of Balance Therapeutics, a division of South Shore Neurologic Associates, P.C., Patchogue, NY. Private Practice: Specializing in the Diagnosis of Disorders of the Vestibular System, Patchogue, NY.

Mitchell Scheiman, O.D., FAAO, FCOVD
Professor of Optometry, Director of Pediatric/Binocular Vision Program, Pennsylvania College of Optometry. Private Practice: Specializing in Rehabilitation Optometry and Vision Therapy in the Philadelphia suburbs.

Irwin B. Suchoff, O.D., D.O.S., FAAO
Distinguished Service Professor Emeritus, State University of New York, State College of Optometry. Founder of that institution's Head Trauma Vision Rehabilitation Unit.

Stacy Trebing, P.T.
Developed and supervised the Vestibular Rehabilitation Service, South Shore Neurologic Associates, Patchogue, NY.

Patricia A. Winkler, M.S., P.T., NCS
Affiliate faculty, Regis University. President, South Valley Physical Therapy, P.D., Englewood, CO.

Dedications

To our families who bore with us through the
editorial process.

To our colleagues of the various rehabilitative professions who contributed to this book.

And to the patients with acquired brain injuries who
taught us so much.

I.B.S.
K.J.C.
N.K.

Acknowledgments

We wish to acknowledge Sally Marshall Corngold whose dedication
and skill in the design and production of this book indicated a labor
of love.
Kathleen Patterson's artistic abilities resulted in the book's cover
which we feel graphically portrays what many people with acquired
brain injury have described to us.
We also wish to acknowledge the contributions made by Dr. Jane
Plass in her excellent job of copyediting and indexing.

An Overview of Acquired Brain Injury and Optometric Implications

Irwin B. Suchoff, O.D., D.O.S.
Neera Kapoor, O.D., M.S.
Kenneth J. Ciuffreda, O.D., Ph.D.

Introduction

Acquired brain injury (ABI) is an umbrella term encompassing those conditions that appear suddenly and result in a neurological dysfunction.[1,2] There are two major precipitating conditions for ABI. See Figure 1. The first is termed traumatic brain injury (TBI) and results from an external insult to the brain. The particular physical event can be classified as a closed or penetrating head injury. Examples of the former are injuries consequent to sports, motor vehicle and industrial accidents. Penetrating head injuries result primarily from gunshots and sharp instruments. A further classification of TBI relates to certain behavioral sequelae at the time of hospitalization, as determined primarily by the Glasgow Coma Scale.[3] This clinical tool quantifies the patient's eye opening, motor, and verbal responsive capabilities into three categories: severe, moderate and mild head injuries.[4] These are useful for the initial characterization of the patient's condition, subsequent monitoring, and prognostication of the long-term life outcome for the patient (Table 1).

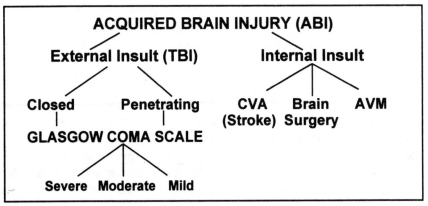

Figure 1. The categories and components of acquired brain injury

Table 1. The Glasgow Coma Scale—Responses and Scoring		
Test	Patient's Response	Assigned Score
Eye Opening	Opens eyes on own	4
	Opens eyes when asked in a loud voice	3
	Opens eyes when pinched	2
	Does not open eyes	1
Motor Response	Follows simple commands	6
	Pulls examiner's hand away when pinched	5
	Pulls part of body away when examiner pinches patient	4
	Flexes body inappropriately to pain (decorticate posturing)	3
	Body becomes rigid in an extended position when examiner pinches victim (decerebrate posturing)	2
	Has no motor response to pinch	1
Verbal Response	Carries on a conversation correctly and tells examiner where he is, who he is, and the month and year	5
	Seems confused or disoriented	4
	Talks so examiner can understand victim but makes no sense	3
	Makes sounds that examiner cannot understand	2
	Makes no sounds	1

Scoring: *Coma–no eye opening, no ability to follow commands, no word verbalizations (3-8)*
Severe head injury–Total score of 8 or less
Moderate head injury–Total score of 9 to 12
Minor head injury–Total score of 13 to 15

Conditions that constitute the second group under ABI result from internally-based brain insults (Figure 1). The most common scenario is a vascular incident, such as ischemic or hemorrhagic stroke (cerebrovascular accident or CVA). However, arteriovenous malformations (AVM) and sequelae of brain surgery are also included. In the remainder of this chapter, CVA will be used to represent the internally-based brain injury category.

Epidemiology

There is general agreement that some 600,000 Americans incur a stroke each year. About 500,000 are first attacks, and the remainder are recurrent attacks.[5] We could not find estimates in our literature search of the incidence of AVMs or ABIs resulting from brain surgery. Consequently, the 600,000 figure is most probably an underestimation of the internal insult category of ABI. The estimated incidence of TBI has varied because there has been a lack of uniform criteria used by different researchers. However, as Elovic and Antoinette point out, the estimate of 200 cases/100,000 population has recently been used in various studies.[6] Thus, with the population of the United States being 270,000,000, [7] some 540,000 Americans incur TBI each year.

There is a difference in age between the two groups. Some 82% who suffer a stroke each year are 65 or older.[5] On the other hand, the highest incidence of TBI is in the 15-24 year age range.[6] Males are the more numerous victims of both stroke and TBI at all ages.[5,6]

Pathophysiology
TBI

In closed-head injuries, there are two types of insult: the acceleration or coup injury occurs when an object in motion, such as a gun or fist, strikes the head, or when a head in motion strikes a stationary hard object. This can result in skull fracture, subdural and epidural hematomas, and contusion to the underlying brain tissue. The deceleration or contrecoup injury occurs after the head is in motion and strikes a stationary object. In automobile accidents, both types of injuries can occur. For example, the force of a rear-end collision causes the head to strike the windshield, resulting in an initial coup injury. Then the sudden deceleration of the head results in a rebound effect and the ensuing contrecoup injury. The brain moves from its usual position, and secondary injury can occur opposite the site of the original injury. Further, rotational forces can cause twisting of the brain. These shearing effects can cause the brain's surface blood vessels to break, thus resulting in hematomas in the epidural or subdural cerebral coverings, in addition to injuries to the brain cell axons (diffuse axonal injury or DAI). Additional damage can be incurred as the brain slides along the rough surfaces of the skull, particularly in the temporal and frontal regions and brain stem (Figure 2).

In penetrating head injury, the damage is less diffuse, since the injury is more focused. Still, a bullet entering a specific area of the brain can impair the subdural and epidural blood vessels and can carry hair and fragments of splintered skull that cause axonal damage and infection. And in both types of TBI, the compromised cerebral blood vessels can result in edema and hematoma, both of which exert pressure on the brain, causing further damage.[8]

Secondary brain injury occurs from hours to several weeks post trauma. The initial trauma disrupts autoregulatory physiologic mechanisms, and neurotoxic compounds are released. There is then a series of biochemical actions which produce free radicals of oxygen. The result is ischemia, thereby producing further damage or destruction of additional brain cells.[8]

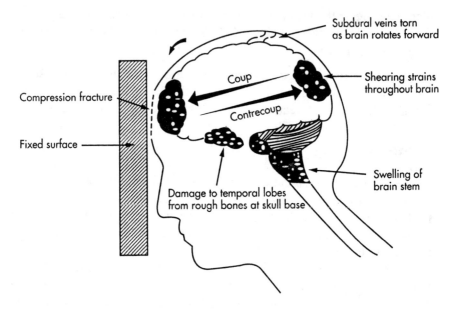

Figure 2. The dynamics of closed-head injury. The coup or acceleration injury occurs when the head hits the fixed surface. The contrecoup or deceleration injury occurs as the head bounces back. Reprinted from Zost, MG. Diagnosis and management of visual dysfunction in cerebral injury. In Maino: DM, ed. Diagnosis and Management of Special Populations. Santa Ana, CA: Optometric Extension Program Foundation, 2001. (Originally published by Mosby.)

CVA

The pathophysiology of CVA is a function of the type (Table 2). When there are physical changes to the arteries sup-

Table 2. Types and Causes of Stroke	
Ischemic	Hemorrhagic
Hypertension Embolism Artherosclerosis	Broken blood vessel Ruptured aneurysm Arteriovenous malformation

plying the brain, ischemia is the consequence. This in turn results in either a localized or diffuse infarction of brain cells, depending on the type of restriction or blockage of the blood vessel. Again, edema follows and exerts pressure on the brain. In hemorrhagic stroke, blood escapes from the vessels with two consequences: areas of the brain distal to the breakage are deprived of oxygen, thereby fostering ischemia. Additionally, pooling of blood in the subarachnoid space causes edema and pressure on the brain itself.[9]

4

Commonalities of TBI and CVA

Thus, there are two distinct subgroups of ABI. The rationale for incorporating the two under ABI is based primarily on the sudden nature of onset, damage to the central nervous system (CNS), and resulting neurological dysfunctions, all of which are common to both. The "suddenness" is arguably the most important factor in understanding these patients. In this context, it is useful to compare ABI to congenital and degenerative conditions that adversely affect the CNS. In congenital conditions, such as fragile X or cerebral palsy, the dysfunctions are there "from the beginning"; in degenerative conditions such as Alzheimer's disease and multiple sclerosis, there is a gradual increase in neurologically-based dysfunctions. In contrast, the ABI patient is one person the moment before the car crash or stroke and a different person afterward. This condition has been termed the "shaken sense of self."[10,11] The resulting psychological, social and fiscal consequences are significant not only to the patient but also to his or her family. Thus, the individual becomes suddenly depressed, cognitively impaired, awkward in social situations, and unable to perform adequately in the workplace.[12]

There are other significant commonalities that the two entities of ABI share. For example, they are served by the same medical care systems. The initial phase requires hospitalization and provides acute care. The practitioner team is most frequently directed by the neurologist, with active participation primarily by the cardiologist, orthopedist and neuro-ophthalmologist. In the subacute care phase, direction becomes increasingly shared with the physiatrist, with occupational, physical, speech and language therapists providing further care along with clinical and neuropsychologists, and sometimes optometrists. In the final phase, rehabilitation, the patient is not always confined to the hospital. However, he or she may return as an outpatient. Other options include seeking these services from appropriate free-standing rehabilitation facilities or from particular independent practitioners. The physiatrist becomes the case manager, and the other medical practitioners serve to maintain the patient's health and well being. Active management and therapy are conducted by the aforementioned professionals, with optometrists recently taking on an increasing role.[13, 14]

The behavioral and functional consequences of CVA are generally less diffuse than in TBI. However, because both categories involve the brain, the sequelae are quite similar. These include attentional, sleep, memory, cognitive and personality disorders in addition to gross and fine motor dysfunctions.[15, 16] Hearing and language disorders (aphasias) are not uncommon,[17,18] along with vestibular disorders resulting in vertigo and balance problems. See the last three chapters of this volume.

Ocular and Visual Sequelae of ABI

Physical damage consequent to TBI can affect any of the structures of the visual system—the orbit, external eye and its associated structures, anterior segment, vitreous, uveal tract, retina, optic nerve, and occipital cortex.[1,19] In CVA, there is usually little injury to the ocular structures. However, there is generally more retinal and crystalline lens pathology from diabetes and hypertension, which are risk factors for CVA. In terms of clinical importance, a recent study reported on 62 ABI patients who had received full optometric evaluations. These individuals were residents at two subacute care facilities, and their brain injuries had occurred at least three years previously. They were examined as part of a general health care program, not necessarily because a visual and/or ocular dysfunction was suspected. The results revealed a significantly higher frequency of dry eye, blepharitis, glaucoma, crystalline lens pathologies, and retinopathies (diabetic and hypertensive) as compared to the non-brain-injured population.[14]

Visual sequelae of TBI and CVA are quite similar. These have been discussed in detail elsewhere.[1,14,20,21] In the study of 62 ABI patients cited above, a high percentage of the subjects manifested binocular fusional deficits, oculomotor dysfunctions and visual field deficits.[14] In our experience, Table 3 is a summary of the most frequent visual dysfunctions that the optometrist or ophthalmologist can expect to be present in the ABI population.

Table 3. Visual Sequelae of ABI

1. Visual field losses—central, congruous and incongruous homonymous hemianopias and quadrantanopias, altitudinal, neglect

2. Eye movement dysfunctions—fixation, pursuit, saccade, nystagmus

3. Ocular muscle dysfunctions—strabismus, anisocoria, lagophthalmus, ptosis

4. Binocular dysfunctions—exophoria, convergence insufficiency, vertical phorias, fusional instabilities

5. Accommodative dysfunctions—amplitude, flexibility, sustainability

6. Perceptual dysfunctions—contrast sensitivity, color vision, body image, left-right discrimination, spatial relationships, agnosias, "subjective visual disturbances," e.g., wavy and shimmering vision, photosensitivity

7. Visually-involved vestibular dysfunctions—vertigo, loss of balance

---

Optometric Implications

It is evident that ocular and visual dysfunctions occur frequently in the ABI population. However, it is not uncommon for these conditions to be overlooked. This is understandable during the acute care phase where the thrust is to keep the individual alive and medically minimize further damage. As the patient enters into a formal program of rehabilitation, these conditions, if unattended, can impede progress and act as an obstacle for the patient to resume normal activities of daily living.[22, 23] Optometry is positioned to meet the ocular and visual needs of these patients. Its history of low vision care and vision therapy has uniquely prepared optometric practitioners to diagnose and manage ABI patients. We propose certain measures to provide optimal care of these individuals.

1. Recognize the functional and behavioral consequences of ABI and make the necessary accommodations. This requires the practitioner to consider the attentional and cognitive sequelae and to allow sufficient time for the examination. The appointment procedure should be designed to ensure that the practitioner is aware, well before the patient arrives, that the patient has incurred ABI. Appointments for these patients should be made for times when the office environment is relatively free of extraneous noise and other distractions. The office should be wheelchair accessible, and appropriate equipment should be available to accommodate aphasic and motor-impaired patients.

2. Be aware of the ocular and visual conditions that are frequently encountered in this population. Since virtually any physical and physiological aspect of the visual system can be adversely affected by ABI, a thorough ocular and vision evaluation is necessary. Special attention should be paid to ocular health, eye movement abilities, binocular motor and sensory functions, accommodative status and visual field integrity.

3. Communicate your findings and their functional consequences to the patient and significant others in a meaningful manner. For example, not infrequently the patient with a binocular dysfunction is aware that "something is wrong" or that "vision gets confused at times." Showing the patient that he is seeing double with a red lens and penlight can be an important step in further treatment. The patient's family can appreciate the condition and resulting confusion by the use of a handheld prism that is sufficient to create diplopia. Another case is when the patient and the family have been told that there is a homonymous hemianopic visual field deficit. Frequently, both patient and family understand this to mean that there is blindness in one eye, e.g., the left eye in a left hemianopia. This can be easily dispelled during visual acuity testing:

the patient can be shown that while he might miss the first several letters of a Snellen line, the ability to discern the remainder of the letters precludes blindness. The family can be shown the functional consequences of the field defect by placing black tape on the left side of each lens of their spectacles (or on a frame with plano lenses) and having them walk down a long hallway or the street.

4. Be aware of and prepared to use all appropriate optometric interventions. These include special considerations for refractive conditions in terms of compensatory lenses; wearing instructions to the patient and involved rehabilitation professionals; frame design and lens type; filtering lenses for photosensitivity; room lighting, compensatory and visual-field-enhancing prisms; vision therapy; and the use of prophylactic and pharmaceutical measures for lid conditions and tear insufficiency.[24]

5. Communicate your findings, treatment plan and recommendations to all other involved rehabilitation professionals. Once the proper release forms have been signed, communication should be conducted in all cases by letters appropriate to the particular professional. Thus, a report to a neurologist or primary care physician should be oriented more toward physical ocular findings and pathologies, while a report to a physiatrist will contain these aspects in addition to the functional implications. Reports to psychologists, occupational therapists and physical therapists should contain the diagnoses but go into more detail as to the functional consequences of their rehabilitation programs. Follow-up communications by telephone serve as progress reports and enhance the ability of all rehabilitation professionals to modify their treatment regimens.

6. Become a proactive member of the rehabilitation team. Seek to join team discussions or grand rounds concerning the patient. Offer to give in-service presentations at meetings of the various professionals on the ocular and visual consequences of ABI and appropriate interventions. Learn to speak the language of the others, and teach them the language of rehabilitation optometry.

References

1. Suchoff IB, Gianutsos R, Ciuffreda KJ, Groffman S. Vision impairment related to acquired brain injury. In: Silverstone B, Lang, MA, Rosenthal BP, Faye EE, eds. The Lighthouse Handbook On Vision Impairment And Vision Rehabilitation, Vol I. New York: Oxford University Press, 2000:549-73.

2. Suchoff IB. Guest editorial. Clinical Eye and Vision Care 1998;10:109-11.

3. Horn LJ, Sherer M. Rehabilitation of traumatic brain injury. In: Grabois M, Garrison SJ, Hart KA, Lehmkul LD, eds. Physical Medicine and Rehabilitation. The Complete Approach. Malden MA: Blackwell Science, 2000:1281-304.

4. Duckett S, Duckett S. The neuropathology of the minor head injury syndrome. In: Mandel S, Sataloff RT, Schapiro SR, eds. Minor Head Trauma Assessment, Management and Rehabilitation. New York: Springer-Verlag, 1993:2-13.

5. American Heart Association. Stroke (brain attack). Available at http://www.americanheart.org/statistics/05stroke.html. Accessed 8/2/99.

6. Elovic E, Antoinette T. Epidemiology and primary prevention of traumatic brain injury. In: Horn LJ, Zasler ND, eds. Medical Rehabilitation of Traumatic Brain Injury. Philadelphia: Hanley & Belfus, 1996:1-28

7. United State Government. People. Available at http://www.odci.gov.cia/publications/factbook/us.html. Accessed 8/2/99.

8. Marion DW. Pathophysiology and initial neurosurgical care: future directions. In: Horn LJ, Zasler ND, eds. Medical Rehabilitation of Traumatic Brain Injury. Philadelphia: Hanley & Belfus, 1996:29-52.

9. Bradshaw JL, Mattingley JB. Clinical Neuropsychology: Behavioral and Brain Science. San Diego: Academic Press, 1995:1-24.

10. Kay T, Newman B, Cavallo M et al. Toward a neuropsychological model of functional disability after mild brain injury. Neuropsychol 1992;6:371-84.

11. Gianutsos R, Suchoff IB. Neuropsychological consequences of mild brain injury and optometric implications. J Behav Optom 1998;1:7-10.

12. Rose CF, Capildeo R. Stroke, the Facts. New York: Oxford Univ. Press, 1981:1-9.

13. Suter PS. A quick start in post-acute vision rehabilitation following brain injury. J Optom Vis Dev 1999; 2:73-82.

14. Suchoff IB, Kapoor N, Waxman R et al. The occurrence of ocular and visual dysfunctions in an acquired brain-injured patient sample. J Am Optom Assoc 1999;5:301-8.

15. Schapiro SR, Sacchetti TS. Neuropsychological sequelae of minor head trauma. In: Mandel S, Sataloff RT, Schapiro SR, eds. Minor Head Trauma Assessment, Management and Rehabilitation. New York: Springer-Verlag, 1993:86-106.

16. Siev E, Freishtat B, Zoltan B. Perceptual and Cognitive Dysfunction in the Adult Stroke Patient. A Manual for Evaluation and Treatment. Thorofare, NJ: Slack, 1986:107-35.

17. Morganstein S, Smith MC. Aphasia and right-hemisphere disorders. In: Gordon WA, ed. Advances in Stroke Rehabilitation. Boston: Andover Medical Publishers, 1993:103-33.

18. Morganstein S, Smith MC. Motor-speech disorders and dysphagia. In: Gordon WA, ed. Advances in Stroke Rehabilitation. Boston: Andover Medical Publishers, 1993:134-61.

19. Vogel M. An overview of head trauma for the primary care practitioner: Part II-ocular damage associated with head trauma. J Am Optom Assoc 1992; 8:542-5.

20. Zost, MG. Diagnosis and management of visual dysfunction in cerebral injury. In: Maino DM, ed. Diagnosis and Management of Special Populations. Santa Ana, CA: Optometric Extension Program Foundation, 2001:75-134. (Originally published by Mosby, 1995.)

21. Cohen AH, Rein LD. The effect of head trauma on the visual system: the doctor of optometry as a member of the rehabilitation team. J Am Optom Assoc 1992;8:530-6.

22. Wainapel SF. Vision rehabilitation: an overlooked subject in physiatric training and practice. Am J Phys Med Rehab 1995;74:313-14.

23. Ciuffreda KJ, Suchoff IB, Kapoor N et al. Normal visual function. In: Gonzalez EG, Myers SJ, Edelstein JF et al, eds. Downey & Darling's Physiological Basis of Rehabilitation Medicine, 3rd edition. Boston: Butterworth-Heinemann, 2001:241-61.

24. Suchoff IB, Gianutsos R. Rehabilitative optometric interventions for the adult with acquired brain injury. In: Grabois M, Garrison SJ, Hart KA et al, eds. Physical Medicine & Rehabilitation. Malden MA: Blackwell Sci, 2000:608-21.

Interdisciplinary Management and Rehabilitation of Acquired Brain-Injured Patients

Edwin F. Richter, III, M.D.

Introduction

Acquired brain injury has been recognized as a major challenge for our health care systems. Advances in acute care methods have led to improved survival rates following major traumatic brain injuries. Educational efforts and outreach programs may improve recognition of minor traumatic brain injuries. These changes may lead to an increase in the previously reported incidence rate of 200 traumatic brain injuries per 100,000 people in the United States.[1,2]

Other types of acquired brain injury have been amenable to risk factor reduction efforts. Stroke has been the third leading cause of death and the leading cause of disability in the United States. Better control of diabetes and hypertension, smoking cessation, and anticoagulation or cardioversion of patients with atrial fibrillation are examples of useful interventions. Working against any favorable trends, however, is the significant increase in stroke risk with age. Public health measures and treatment of other conditions have allowed more people to survive to geriatric age brackets. This puts more people at risk for stroke. Future advances in treating comorbidities after acute stroke may also result in more disabled stroke survivors.

The social implications of brain injury are not fully conveyed by incidence rates. Traumatic brain injury is a major source of disability in young adults. Men have traditionally been at significantly higher risk, but increasing participation by women in dangerous occupations and sports will likely reduce this disparity. Although there is also a rise in traumatic brain injury incidence after age 60, the economic impact is particularly severe when young people become disabled. Loss of earning potential combines with costs of care across potentially long life spans in such cases. Total cost to society in 1985 was estimated at $37.8 billion.[3] More recently, this has been estimated to be $48.3 billion.[4] Aside from the economic impact, the burden of care placed on families should be considered. Beyond direct expenditures, caregivers lose vocational or avocational opportunities, with potential adverse effects on their quality of life.

There are many types of disabling conditions. Acquired brain injury has particularly problematic aspects. Cognitive and behavioral changes are particularly disruptive. Modern technology, traditional assistive devices, and barrier-free design can partially reduce the impact of physical impairments.[5] Social and political activism has lowered some legal and economic obstacles for the disabled.[6] These interventions have been helpful for brain injury survivors, but their complex array of impairments, disabilities, and handicaps poses problems beyond those faced by other patient populations. Mentation deficits or emotional changes may hinder utilization of resources that amputees or paraplegics might find beneficial. These factors will tend to keep the burden of care for significant others and for society at large relatively high.

Given these problems, any reasonable approach to enhancing current methods of care should be considered. Realistically, economic factors require that any proposal for change be likely to prove cost-effective. Plans that require any major increase in health care costs would be unlikely to be implemented, even if there is a good chance of achieving later savings or other benefits to society. This creates a need for models of care that do not rely on increased funding for rehabilitation.

One such model is an interdisciplinary approach, in which involved professionals go beyond narrow concepts of compartmentalized treatment to share expertise and understanding across traditional boundaries. Better communication and coordination of care should then potentiate utilization of existing resources.

True interdisciplinary evaluation and treatment should go well beyond concurrent involvement of professionals from multiple disciplines on a case. Team members need formal and informal lines of effective communication. To avoid conflicts and enhance their own effectiveness, they should learn from colleagues about how the other disciplines approach clinical problems. At times, two or more team members may treat a patient together in a formal cotreatment session. More commonly, treatment plans for a given time period are coordinated to reinforce certain themes and promote consistent behavior. Avoidance of mixed messages is a priority.

This philosophy is not always instilled during professional training. Clinical training is usually provided by educators from that particular profession. Expertise within their fields and loyalty to the worthy ideals of relevant professional organizations do not automatically prepare clinicians for interdisciplinary work. Even within a profession or specialty, collegiality between individuals or subspecialties may not be given much formal emphasis during training. Clinicians with overlapping areas of expertise may view each other as competitors. Old resentments and institutional rivalries may pose barriers to change.

However, other factors have encouraged professionals interested in interdisciplinary concepts. Successful collaboration on isolated cases may lead to discussions about the rehabilitation process. Organizations that attract members of multiple professions provide further opportunities for interaction. Some teaching institutions do recruit guest lecturers and promote interdisciplinary conferences.

In recent years, concepts of rehabilitation teams have been explored in the professional literature.[7] Interprofessional relationships and treatment effectiveness have been explored. Skilled clinicians still have good reason to question whether they need to invest the time and effort to adapt to interdisciplinary approaches. Any substantial change in practice habits requires justification. A fuller appreciation of the problems faced across various other disciplines, linked with increased awareness of how rehabilitation teams might function, could lead to further interest in this type of activity.

Selected Rehabilitation Problems
Specific conditions

Awareness and understanding of medical problems are generally recognized as priorities in contemporary biopsychosocial and consumer-based treatment models. An informed patient can participate more effectively in making decisions. Understanding current problems and potential for change must precede any realistic setting of goals. Plans should then be based on those goals. This process should include a realistic assessment of available resources. When several goals can be identified, relative importance and feasibility may drive decisions regarding allocation of finite resources, including the patient's time and energy.

Cognitive deficits and behavioral disorders are obstacles to optimal patient involvement in planning and decision making. Severely injured patients may lack the ability to comprehend even basic issues. Highly agitated patients may even pose danger to themselves or others. Initial acute care of these patients follows a traditional medical model. Reduction of adverse stimuli, medication management and, when necessary, limited use of restraints are among the available interventions. On a brain injury unit, behavioral approaches may be employed effectively.[8] Careful clinical judgment is needed to determine how much activity and stimulation can be tolerated in these circumstances. Maintaining a quiet environment, limiting visitors, and incorporating rest breaks into a program may be indicated. Potentially beneficial therapies may have to be introduced slowly at this stage. Even patients with decreased arousal levels may prove susceptible to excessive stimulation.

Patients who appear relatively normal may still have significant deficits. Difficulty with initiation may leave them dependent on others for cueing. Attention and concentration deficits may cause rapid deterioration of performance of a task that may initially be approached adequately. Distractibility may reflect inability to suppress awareness of background stimuli while attending to a task. Various types of memory deficit may hinder storage or recall of recent information. Impulsiveness reduces effectiveness of sensory integration, motor performance and higher level intellectual tasks. Rigid, inflexible cognitive styles, with difficulty shifting between topics or changing strategies, may cause a tendency to "get stuck" and perseverate over a problem. Strategies learned in one context may not be carried over into other relevant situations. The relevance may not be perceived, or initiation may not be adequate to launch the strategy. Any combination of these disorders may prevent multitasking. Success at a given activity may require an optimal environment, and it may come with the inability to sustain further effective cognitive efforts. Loss of mental endurance is less easily measured than inability to walk beyond a given distance, but it is arguably of greater functional significance.

Emotional disorders are not always easily separated from cognitive deficits following brain injury. Disturbance of emotional status can certainly impair performance, even in the absence of brain injury. Susceptibility may, however, be much greater in some brain injury survivors. In some cases, we may be able to speculate about anatomical locations of injury within the brain. For example, my experience indicates that lesions within the limbic system may change behavior patterns; the septum pallucidum has been associated with aspects of behavior, including rage; the amygdala (anatomically part of the basal ganglia) appears to play a role in control of socially appropriate behavior; frontal lesions can cause loss of ability to impose higher level emotional control, in addition to intellectual deficits. Given our limited knowledge of the complex interactions between structures within the brain, we cannot point with great certainty to specific locations of pathology in many of our patients. In some cases, behavioral changes may be direct consequences of brain injury. In other cases, emotional responses to either the injury or the resulting disability may be problematic. Such responses do not occur in a vacuum, and interactions with other people and institutions add other layers of complexity to the problem.

Communication disorders can magnify the scope of any cognitive or emotional problems. Disorders of language skills, such as aphasia, can interfere with both expressive and receptive functions. Articulation deficits can make speech less intelligible. A concurrent upper extremity motor deficit may hinder writing, using a keyboard, or even pointing at pictures. Iatrogenic factors, such as endotracheal intubation, may also interfere. Premorbid status also should be considered. Patients who had not previously learned the language of their present society and of their health care providers are at an obvious disadvantage. Those who had become fluent in that language as an adult may have a significant loss of that ability after certain brain injuries and may benefit from interaction in whatever language they retain the best.

Auditory dysfunction may occur as a result of some brain injuries. Other patients may have been compensating for partial hearing loss before their brain injuries occurred. They may not have been consciously aware of the problem but were able to attend closely to others speaking to them. Their ability to compensate may be reduced by the brain injury.

Eating and swallowing are functions that are usually given little conscious thought. Various problems may arise after brain injury. Impaired sense of smell (usually from injury to cranial nerve I) is more likely to occur than loss of ability to taste, but either can decrease appetite. Poor coordination of swallowing (dysphagia) can lead to aspiration pneumonia. Clinical assessment can be enhanced by studies like videoflouroscopy, which observe the swallowing of different textures dynamically. Restrictions on certain textures of foods, especially thin liquids, may allow safe adequate oral nutrition. If not, then a feeding tube is indicated. A nasogastric tube is often not well tolerated for long. It can be replaced by percutaneous endoscopic gastrostomy (PEG), in which a tube is placed through an opening in the abdominal wall. The procedure is relatively low risk, allows oral intake to continue as tolerated, and is reversible. It does not replace the emotional satisfaction of eating.

The patient's nutritional status is usually altered after brain injury. Perceptions of hunger, thirst, or satiety may be altered. Disinhibition may reduce control of eating or drinking. In the hospital, procedures and tests may interfere with meal delivery. Containers and utensils may be hard to manipulate. For the ambulatory outpatient, memory or performance deficits may interfere with maintaining adequate intake.

Administration of medications is a potential barrier to independent living. Complex regimens are easy to initiate in the acute care setting. They are more difficult in a rehabilitation center, since patients must attend therapies during the day. In a home setting, certain regimens may prove too complex. This is a particular concern with insulin-dependent diabetics. Testing blood sugar via finger-stick, drawing up the correct amount of insulin into a syringe, and injecting it may be too difficult for many different reasons.

Seizure control is another medical concern. About 5% of patients are anticipated to develop post-traumatic epilepsy.[9] Medication compliance and avoidance of risky activities, such as driving, are important issues. Avoiding stimuli that might trigger seizure activity is important for some patients, such as those whose seizures can be induced by flickering lights from a video game screen or sunlight viewed while riding in a car past a picket fence. In some cases, the signs of seizure activity are quite subtle and may initially be overlooked or misdiagnosed.

Vestibular dysfunction is relatively common after head injury, even in the absence of skull fractures. Some patients who are clinically suspected of having seizures are later found to have vestibular deficits. Benign paroxysmal positional vertigo is probably the most common form, and it responds relatively well to postural maneuvers. Central lesions are more difficult to treat, but are reported to respond to gaze stabilization exercises and balance exercises.[10] Patients with visual or somatosensory deficits would be expected to have more difficulty compensating for vestibular balance disorders.

Not all brain-injured patients will give clear complaints of dizziness and/or vertigo. Partial synonyms, such as "light-headed" or "floating," may be recognized by a clinician and further explored. Testing of the ability to stand with eyes open or shut with feet together (Romberg test) or with either foot directly in front of the other (sharpened Romberg) can be done without special equipment. Clinical suspicion can justify referral for balance platform testing or electronystagmography. These tests can provide objective measurements of vestibular system function. Balance platform testing may also reveal patterns that suggest efforts to simulate pathology, such as sinusoidal patterns of sway. Measurements may also be used to document progress during treatment.

Balance problems may be multifactorial. Humans rely on visual, vestibular, and somatosensory input to determine their position. A deficiency in any one of these areas may impair balance, although the systems are sufficiently complementary that under favorable conditions good compensation is possible. Adequate motor strength is needed to maintain stability during dynamic activity. Injury to the cerebellum may cause ataxia with defective coordination. Involvement of the basal ganglia may hinder aspects of motor performance. Sensory deficits, from either central injuries or concurrent peripheral nerve pathology, will limit awareness of body position. Patients with balance deficits are at increased risk for falls, which can lead to additional injuries. The level of risk can be predicted from quantitative measures, such as the Berg balance scale. Observation of performance in real-life settings (or realistic simulations) may also help detect risk factors for additional injuries. Aside from the concern that such injuries could further impair performance, the potential effects of recurrent falls on a patient's morale should not be underestimated.

Ocular and visual problems are frequent sequelae of acquired brain injury.[11] Diseases such as glaucoma or damage to the ocular structure are most often recognized in the acute care setting. However, more subtle subsequent dysfunctions of the oculomotor, accommodative and visual perceptual systems most frequently are not detected. A clear and succinct complaint of diplopia and/or photophobia is occasionally volunteered, but more typically, any clues to the presence of visual dysfunction are offered in the form of problems with functional tasks. Fatigue or headaches during reading are nonspecific complaints that could lead to discovery of significant underlying problems. Preliminary findings of visual field cuts or convergence deficits are examples of abnormalities that warrant further exploration. Observation of nystagmus may be significant, but this may be seen routinely in any patient who is taking phenytoin (Dilantin). One would like to obtain a good premorbid history of visual function, but since many patients had little formal evaluation before their brain injuries, the only alternative is to review any indirect evidence. Screening during school programs, during pre-employment physical examinations, or during application for a driver's license is usually limited to minimal testing of visual acuity in standard conditions. Previous ability to perform certain types of vocational or recreational activities may reveal more about premorbid function.

Clinical considerations
Testing done in relatively favorable conditions may not reflect all the problems that ensue in other situations. Controlled levels of ambient light and/or noise may be critical for some patients. Other patients may pay special attention to their needs for adequate rest and nutrition before scheduled evaluations but neglect these at other times. This apparent noncompliance is not necessarily willful refusal to follow instructions, as many patients simply do not have adequate resources available to them. The presence of a supportive professional in a secure environment may reduce anxiety. Such a clinical setting can encourage conscious attention to any strategies previously learned, even before specific instructions are given. A desire to please a treating clinician may motivate a level of effort that cannot be consistently sustained over a longer period. Any combination of these factors could lead to deceptively high levels of achievement during formal testing.

An individual's performance may vary significantly at times for a variety of legitimate reasons. Fatigue may cause some brain-injured patients to show a marked deterioration of performance during the course of their day. Fluctuations in emotional state may cause equally severe but less predictable changes. Brain injury survivors may be more susceptible than other patients to difficulties when working with individuals with whom they have suboptimal interpersonal relationships. Different treatment sites may have environmental factors that impact their well-being. Even the way patients commute to treatment areas may influence their conditions. Aside from generally making their lives more difficult, these phenomena may cause treatment staff seeing them at different times to form different opinions of their abilities, cooperation or motivation.

When any professional evaluates a patient and reaches conclusions that are markedly inconsistent with the opinions of other professionals, then careful attention must be paid to the situation. Within a given specialty, there are of course different levels of general expertise and practical experience with particular problems. There can also be honest differences of opinion between comparably proficient experts, especially in clinical conditions where judgment calls are required in the lack of universally accepted "gold standard" diagnostic criteria. In certain settings, questions may also be raised about the professional's self-interest. Issues such as compensation, prestige, need for research subjects or teaching cases, and desire to please interested parties may be debated.

Different specialists within the same profession may take very different approaches to patients. Often definite benefits derive from this, since specialist expertise may be needed for many different problems. It would be naïve, for example, to think that one physician should handle all the problems of a severely injured patient without drawing upon the skills of available consultants. The regular primary care physician might initially be unaware of the patient's arrival at an emergency room and therefore would need to update the situation after trauma specialists initiated a care plan. Neurosurgeons, neurologists, and a wide array of other consultants may be needed. They would be expected to focus on their areas of expertise, although there are areas of overlap. Decisions on how to prioritize treatment of different problems may require discussion. By convention, the service that admits the patient is expected to coordinate this process, although active involvement of the primary care physician can greatly facilitate planning. (In recent years, "hospitalists" and "intensivists" who work exclusively with acute inpatients have begun taking some of that responsibility from office-based practitioners.)

Without minimizing the challenges of making acute care decisions, it is fair to say that patients and families may begin to hear the most conflicting recommendations when rehabilitation issues are introduced. Some acute care specialists may have little formal training in rehabilitation, which may contribute to overly optimistic or pessimistic opinions about what may be done. Physicians also vary greatly in their willingness to make predictions. In some cases, it appears convenient to forecast that a severely disabled patient will make a great recovery after rehabilitation, hoping that any angry or frustrated responses may then be delayed until the patient has left the acute care setting. In that situation, a family may focus on advice that therapy must be "aggressive" and needs to start immediately. They may later conclude that undesirable outcomes reflected failure to do therapy quickly enough or vigorously enough. Experienced rehabilitation staff will have difficulty convincing them that pushing a patient beyond appropriate limits is harmful and unethical. This may lead to scenarios where relatives bring in college textbooks to quiz patients who cannot comprehend basic conversations or drag obtunded patients out of bed in disastrous attempts to force them to walk. These events lead to further confrontations with staff, polarizing relationships. Ironically, doctors who made wildly optimistic predictions at earlier stages of care may be remembered fondly as having positive attitudes, while later attempts at realistic counseling are viewed as sadistic. A careful balance must be struck between taking away hope and perpetuating denial.

Early involvement of physiatrists, who specialize in physical medicine and rehabilitation, at the acute care facility can help to make initially sound decisions regarding rehabilitation and realistic expectations of outcomes. The physiatrist should also guide the direction of patients to the most appropriate next level of care, which might be acute inpatient rehabilitation, subacute care, nursing home care, home care, or outpatient therapy. This can still be quite difficult if mixed messages are being sent by other specialists.

Other factors may lead to overly hopeful attitudes. The public is often dazzled by media accounts of medical advances. Even serious journalists and ethical medical experts may inadvertently raise popular expectations too high. In an increasingly competitive health care industry, even conservative providers have begun advertising, as well as seeking increased media coverage for successful programs and new technologies. Around-the-clock availability of data via Internet sources has exponentially increased the ability of computer users to access vast amounts of information, without necessarily enhancing their ability to interpret it. Celebrities who announce their determination to overcome brain injuries or related disorders display courage, heighten awareness, and help fundraising for research, but their cases may be very different than those who seek to emulate them.

This review of the rehabilitation problems and clinical considerations associated with acquired brain injuries, while extensive, is by no means exhaustive. There is also a broad spectrum of comorbidities that may complicate any case. Either pre-existing conditions or complications of the injury may create obstacles to treatment. These add to the challenges faced by the treating clinician and should be appreciated by subsequent rehabilitation professionals.

Rehabilitation Teams

As noted above, physiatrists and nurses are members of the treatment teams at rehabilitation hospitals. Typical inpatient rehabilitation teams also include, as appropriate to the individual case, physical therapists, occupational therapists, speech therapists (speech and language pathologists and swallowing disorder specialists), psychologists, social workers, recreation therapists, vocational rehabilitation counselors, dieticians, orthotists, pharmacists, and chaplains. Consultants from other disciplines, such as optometrists, may be called in as needed. When equipment is ordered, company representatives or equipment dealers may also become involved.

Physiatrist

A physiatrist is a physician specializing in the rehabilitation of disabled individuals. Physiatrists usually serve as the primary attending physician for patients admitted to rehabilitation hospitals. At a minimum, training for the specialty includes one year of internship and three years of residency. The training includes special emphasis on medical problems of disabled populations, as well as rehabilitation strategies and techniques. Diagnosis of relevant conditions, prevention of complications, and reduction of risk factors are among the priorities instilled. Medications, therapies, and devices may be ordered within the rehabilitation care plan. Many physiatrists also learn special procedures, including injections to reduce pain or spasticity.

In addition to learning medical management skills, a physiatrist is responsible for learning team leadership skills. Traditional acute medical care involves individual conversations and written communication among physicians, nurses, and, in some situations, technicians. The complexities of inpatient rehabilitation have long necessitated more formal team conferences. Formats may vary, but flow of information among disciplines should be achieved. Pursuit of this goal must often be weighed against time constraints. Team members who are familiar with their colleagues' abilities and practice patterns should be able to make better use of these opportunities. The physiatrist is expected to maintain open active lines of communication.

Physical therapist

For brain-injured patients, physical therapy may include exercise, ranging of joints, and facilitation of motor recovery. Bed mobility and transfer skills (moving between beds, chairs, toilets, etc.) are addressed. These lessons are followed by balance exercises and gait training. Application of modalities (heat, cold, ultrasound, electrical, etc.) may reduce pain or facilitate mobility. There is an important educational component. Patients and their caregivers are trained to perform an increasing number of exercises and activities. Since treatment time is finite, the expectation is that skills and techniques will be carried over into a daily routine.

Some physical therapists have special training in treating vestibular disorders. Their work includes balance retraining and vestibular habituation exercises. Increasing the vestibular system's tolerance of stressful conditions can lead to important gains in comfort and safety. Assignment of exercises to practice between sessions leads to eventual ability to carry on with a home program.

Driver education is another important area for physical and/or occupational therapists. Some urban areas do have adequate, safe and accessible public transportation systems, but in many parts of this country, loss of the ability to drive is quite limiting. Social isolation is not the least of the potential consequences. Suitable candidates can be tested initially in simulated settings. Later, in actual road tests in vehicles with dual controls, patients drive with the instructor. Various team members may contribute to this aspect of rehabilitation. Factors such as ability to read signs or control emotions may be evaluated. Counseling about avoiding even moderate alcohol intake or certain types of driving conditions may be appropriate. In contemporary practice, most actual driver training is done on an outpatient basis, but the fundamental processes can start with inpatients. Establishing the ability to transfer into a car safely is an example of such an inpatient intervention.

Occupational therapist

Occupational therapy may also include upper extremity exercise, ranging, facilitation, and splinting. Some interventions may be preventive, such as providing orthoses to prevent contractures. Others are adaptive, such as training patients to use reachers, long-handled shoehorns, and sock pullers to substitute for physical abilities that have become restricted. Restorative interventions include exercises to increase strength and coordination. Occupational therapists provide retraining in performance of functional tasks and activities of daily living. They teach use of adaptive equipment. Home management may require significant change of old habits, with emphasis on safety and attention to specific tasks. Basic cognitive and perceptual retraining may be needed before the patient's personal goals can be pursued. This unfortunately may involve making some deficits evident to patients who have been unable or unwilling to recognize problems. Persuading formerly successful individuals that they need to write down even the most mundane information in a notebook or daily planner can be a major undertaking. Convincing patients with combinations of visual field cuts and hemisensory neglect that they must scan their meal tray before complaining that no fork was provided can be difficult. Concerted team interventions may be needed to help patients tolerate the distress they experience as such difficulties are encountered.

Prevocational training is another potential role for occupational therapists. Before formal vocational evaluations are performed, attention can be paid to basic skills that will affect vocational potential. Devices such as ergometers can reproduce some physical workplace challenges. Assigning tasks to be done in noisy environments addresses another potential functional issue. Ability to maintain attention and susceptibility to fatigue can be measured.

Some occupational therapists specialize in electronic technical aids. Increasing availability of computer technology expands human potential. Modified keyboards, joysticks, light pens, and other devices make computers more accessible. Voice recognition technology further minimizes the need for manual skills. Programs with helpful prompts reduce the impact of decreased memory. Therapy "homework" can be done on computers, extending the efficiency of treatment. Connection to the Internet opens lines of interactive communication for even homebound or institutionalized patients. Environmental control units allow greater control of household appliances.

Swallowing disorder treatment plans often draw upon the expertise of multiple disciplines. Most often speech therapists teach swallowing exercises and compensatory techniques, but in some institutions, occupational therapists take responsibility for this area. In either case, occupational therapists still contribute to the care plan through their work, training patients how to eat independently once again. Nurses monitor and reinforce compliance with these lessons and observe for signs of aspiration. Dieticians must ensure that nutritional needs are met, while trying to provide reasonably appealing meals that comply with necessary precautions. Physiatrists must coordinate this process, promote patient and family compliance, order further diagnostic testing as needed, and intervene if problems arise. Input from otolaryngologists, gastroenterologists, pulmonologists, and infectious disease specialists may be requested and coordinated.

Speech and language pathologist

Speech and language pathologists evaluate many other important functions. Effective speech must be loud enough and clear enough for the listener to receive information. More subtle problems include deficiencies of rate control, ability to modulate tone and volume to convey emotional states and conform to social norms, and monitoring of a listener's responses while speaking. A fixed vocal volume deficit may be corrected with amplification, but articulation and prosody problems will not be helped at all. Computerized speech synthesizers allow even mute patients to communicate audibly, if they can operate the system adequately. Otherwise, the output is, at least currently, in a monotone. Treatment approaches may be guided by input from otolaryngologic assessment, including fiber optic visualization of the vocal cords. Effective therapy through voice exercises and articulation retraining requires ongoing practice. Supporting patient motivation is therefore essential.

Language disorders may be more disabling than mechanical speech production problems. Vocal cord paralysis by itself would not preclude effective listening or writing, but damage to the language center may take away these functions in addition to interfering with verbal output. Impaired comprehension may also hinder ability to understand explanations of what has happened or how to proceed. Patients struggling to communicate may become angry with themselves or listeners. Frustration may discourage further attempts to improve performance. These responses can lead to increasing social isolation and disrupt the whole treatment plan. Addressing these issues is an important aspect of speech therapy.

Other areas of concern include the misperceptions of some other professionals, who may mistake communication disorders for global losses of all cognitive functions. That error could lead to withholding other appropriate treatment. Assumptions that these patients are deliberately refusing to follow instructions or answer questions, when in fact there is a lack of ability to understand adequately, could lead to inappropriate clinical management in many areas. Understanding how individual patients are performing in speech therapy can help prevent such errors. Speech pathologists can provide such information, while also raising other team members' general understanding of communication disorders.

Rehabilitation psychologist

Rehabilitation psychologists (clinical and neuropsychological) may perform extensive batteries of cognitive tests. These may include measures of general information, attention, concentration, spatial organization, perception, cognitive flexibility, and memory functions. These are compared to established norms. Interpretation is done with attention to age, education, and vocational history.

In the initial stages of inpatient rehabilitation, most brain-injured patients do not have the stamina to undergo every potentially relevant neuropsychological test. A significant aphasia may preclude meaningful administration of any language-dependent measures. Impaired vision may also hinder evaluation via standard tests. Aside from any new visual deficits from a brain injury, some patients present with premorbid conditions that were not optimally treated. Others may now be unable to report that they lost their reading glasses or left them at home, causing unfortunate delays in treatment. Bedside assessments are sometimes hindered by the distractions of surrounding hospital activities.

These factors necessitate development of practical screening intakes, which allow reasonably fast and accurate evaluations of important aspects of function. These findings will help guide further stages of testing. Meanwhile, the psychologist must inform the rehabilitation team of the preliminary findings. The presence of cognitive or perceptual deficits may explain numerous types of performance problems. This information should be used to direct treatment strategies, such as how new concepts are presented or behaviors are reinforced.

This understanding of why certain practical problems occur should also be conveyed to patients and families as clearly as possible. Organic brain dysfunction may otherwise be interpreted as a lack of motivation. Difficulty performing previously routine tasks might be mistakenly attributed to other coincidental issues. As cognitive testing uncovers pathological findings, explanations of their clinical significance are warranted to improve understanding of the practical issues at hand. Areas of preserved ability should also be highlighted. Aside from potentially boosting morale, this also helps promote understanding of treatment approaches that tap into these areas of relative strength.

Shorter lengths of stay, staffing patterns, need for other treatments, and other practical considerations impose limits on the amount of formal cognitive retraining done on acute inpatient services. Creative responses to this problem include recruiting other team members, who incorporate aspects of cognitive retraining into their routine interactions with patients. Reinforcing orientation and utilization of written schedules are examples of simple interactions that help the pursuit of inpatient treatment goals. These interventions are expected to lead to further carryover at later stages of care.

Psychosocial interventions may be of more acute significance than formal cognitive retraining sessions in earlier stages of recovery. Emotional distress can greatly reduce performance skills. Depression and anxiety reduce ability to participate effectively in treatment. This linkage between emotional state and performance sets up a potential downward spiral of worsening mood and failure to meet objective goals. Helping patients and families avoid this pitfall is a team responsibility, with particular need for the efforts of psychologists and social workers. For some religious patients, coordinated involvement of pastoral care staff may prove particularly appropriate. No single formula covers all facets of enhancing emotional well-being, and input from any team member may prove useful.

Social worker
Social workers help patients face many important practical issues. Most immediately, insurance coverage for rehabilitation varies widely among different commercial or managed care plans. Regulations governing Medicaid, workers' compensation, and no fault insurance programs vary by state. Medicare regulations may be interpreted differently by various regional agencies. As a rule, it is currently more difficult to obtain coverage for services than it was in previous decades. More criteria must be met to get any coverage, and the period for which coverage is authorized tends to be much shorter than what was formerly allowed. These trends are particularly challenging for brain-injured individuals, given the need to quickly process the complexities of these financial issues. Even the most supportive families may be so overwhelmed by other issues that they are at a disadvantage when addressing coverage issues. They benefit from the guidance of a resourceful professional who understands the technical details of their financial concerns and the psychosocial impact of the situation.

Any need for further care at subacute or long-term care facilities raises a variety of concerns. How to pay for such care is perhaps the most obvious pragmatic question, but other deeper worries also arise. At a minimum, a recommendation from a rehabilitation team to transfer to such a facility indicates that a return to home will be delayed. Doubts about ever returning home also arise. The fear of permanently residing in a nursing home is strongly expressed by many individuals. Aside from reservations about the nature of such facilities, there are concerns about what such a development indicates about their relationships with their significant others or their status in society. Some Americans are very conscious of their ethnic cultural heritage but lack practical access to the family or community resources that in other places or times might have facilitated care at home. This deviation from their ideals adds another layer of distress to a difficult situation.

Ability to return home may hinge on how much help is available. Most insurance programs provide only a few hours of attendant care per day, plus occasional visits by a nurse, for a finite period. This may come as a surprise to those who assume that any reasonable health care need will always be covered. The reality is that assistance with dressing, grooming, hygiene, household chores, and shopping is often defined as custodial care. Rehabilitation social workers help organize appropriate resources for patients based on a team's evaluation of their needs. This may involve realistic appraisal of a family's ability to hire help or take on tasks themselves. Identification of other resources, such as government programs or community organizations, is then pursued.

Recreational therapist
Recreational needs may seem less consequential when weighed against the daunting problems noted above. Clinicians must remember that they are not repairing mechanical devices. Recreational therapy not only improves morale, but also provides exposure to situations where recently regained abilities can be applied. This positive reinforcement may be more potent than that provided in traditional clinical settings. Recreational therapists can add significant value to a team.

Dietician
Nutritional needs also deserve significant emphasis. Patients often arrive at a rehabilitation setting with clinical and laboratory evidence of nutritional deficiencies. Potential causes include difficulty handling utensils, poor appetite, or swallowing problems. Prior dietary habits must also be considered. A dietician can help address these issues by working with other team members. Physicians may also prescribe medications to improve appetite or enhance nutritional status. The question of how nutritional needs are to be met after discharge to home often demands sound interdisciplinary coordination. Budgeting, shopping, and safe performance of kitchen activities are just a few of the issues that may require team interventions.

Vocational rehabilitation counselor
Vocational concerns lead to involvement of rehabilitation counselors. In early stages, their role may be more informational. Important early interventions include reviewing vocational history and interests, initiation of contact with employers when appropriate, and referrals to government or voluntary agencies. Later interventions include more intensive counseling,

diagnostic vocational evaluations, and work site placements. Brain-injured individuals with some potential to return to the workforce may at some point also have to weigh the risks of losing coverage under Medicare or Medicaid, as well as disability payments.

Eyecare professions

In most institutionally-based rehabilitative settings, a neuro-ophthalmologist is available for consultations. However, optometrists, who are skilled in the rehabilitation of the ocular and visual sequelae of acquired brain injury, are not usually staff in inpatient subacute or rehabilitation programs. This limits the rehabilitation initiatives commonly provided for vision problems in that setting. Thus, scanning techniques for visual field defects and patching to eliminate diplopia are used, although the application of yoked and compensatory prism that optometrists commonly provide, might well be more effective treatment modalities.

At present, the lack of on-site availability to inpatients is one factor hindering involvement of optometrists. Another is the lack of familiarity of many rehabilitation professionals with the types of vision evaluation and rehabilitation that can be provided. Consequently, initiation of such care is sometimes deferred until after discharge. This may require the optometrist to evaluate the patient without much information about the inpatient stay. Integration of the optometrist's care into the overall treatment plan in these instances presents a significant challenge.

As noted previously, there are many types of professionals routinely included in traditional rehabilitation teams. This review has thus far included several disciplines that are frequently involved in the care of patients with brain injuries. These brief summaries of activities associated with these disciplines are by no means exhaustive. It is hoped that a sense of the various challenges faced by these team members is evident.

Outpatient Issues

Outpatients may face more fragmented care than inpatients for several reasons. Some receive care at home from agency personnel, whose only contact with the referring physician may be through notes sent in the mail. Many nurses and therapists who work in that setting make special efforts to coordinate care, but the logistics may be difficult. Other patients may pursue outpatient treatment at multiple venues. They may need to change providers when their insurance coverage changes. They may see multiple physicians, who in turn send them for different types of therapy. They may grow frustrated with certain providers, leading to changes within a team or change of the entire team.

Some situations do warrant a change of treatment personnel. Even with the best of intentions, the relationship between a clinician and patient may not be conducive to the best possible outcome. Seeking specialist expertise or a fresh perspective may also justify a change of personnel within a center or even changing treatment centers. The concern is that some patients or families "shop" for providers without ever settling down to work with anyone. This can be a way of avoiding unpleasant realities. If they do eventually accept that there is no "big professor" somewhere with a definitive cure, they may find that they have wasted considerable time and money. They may also have missed opportunities for reasonable treatment approaches.

Patients who seek concurrent care from specialists separated by geography or philosophy also risk receiving fragmented care. A distinguished expert at a remote location may offer useful insights, but would not be in an ideal position to provide daily management of care. An orthopedist and a neurologist may suggest different etiologies for a patient's headaches, such as cervicogenic factors versus migraines. Both physicians may disagree with injections recommended by an anesthesiologist, and the patient may wind up with three different sets of medication. Disastrous drug interactions may follow this scenario. In other settings, an essential medication may be stopped on the advice of an unconventional practitioner. This decision may not be reported to the prescribing physician, who might then make other treatment decisions without this important information.

Other contradictions may develop within an institution's treatment plan if the team is not coordinated. A speech pathologist may disagree with the utilization of tests that are heavily dependent on language skills for certain patients. Ideally, this would be addressed on a programmatic level, so that the institution would promote a rational approach to the evaluation of patients with linguistic deficits. On an individual level, early recommendations to colleagues could prevent inappropriate testing or treatments. If each discipline works in relative isolation, then the patient will not benefit from such input.

In recent years, closer involvement of managed care organizations has posed another set of challenges for outpatient programs. Some plans may require that all treatment be done within a given period. Others may offer a finite number of treatment sessions, thus forcing providers and patients to decide how to allocate visits across disciplines. Treatment by psychologists may be considered a mental health issue, leading to more limited coverage. Cognitive rehabilitation may be denied by carriers who consider such treatment similar to long-term psychoanalysis. Other patients who need better pain control or enhanced vision before they can really benefit from intensive cognitive retraining may find that their coverage has been exhausted.

Interdisciplinary Solutions

Certain realities must be recognized. Resources are likely to remain limited by financial constraints. Professionals will have a natural tendency to consider their interventions to be particularly important. Brain injury survivors will face difficulties navigating through complex health care systems.

A genuine commitment to interdisciplinary solutions requires formation of treatment teams that can establish effective modes of communication. Respect for others' expertise is essential. Willingness to go beyond narrow definitions of roles allows better collaboration. Clinicians must be alert for signs of problems that a colleague might be able to address, as well as those traditionally treated by their own discipline. Willingness to monitor for compliance with another therapist's program extends the team's reach. Presenting a united front on major themes, such as the importance of steady attendance and completion of homework, amplifies these messages.

Patients benefit from a clear perception that their treatment team communicates effectively. When one clinician refers to a colleague's findings and recommendations, the implicit respect reinforces the importance of the information. Patients also appreciate that team members care enough about their case to hold discussions or review reports. Since therapists may appear to be working on discrete issues, patients may otherwise fear that their care is fragmented. If they know that their speech problems have been reviewed with all team members, they may have reduced fears of being misunderstood by everyone but the speech pathologist. They also may better trust the team's consensus on how much time to allocate for treatment of different problems.

A perception that the team has a reasonable degree of consensus on plans and goals benefits patients in various ways. Overall respect for the clinicians may be increased. Given that they may receive information about many other types of treatment, including some of dubious value, this may help patients focus on their current regimen. While we should be candid about limitations of the current state of the art, there is still a need to instill confidence to facilitate compliance. If attainable short-term goals were set after initial evaluations, then such confidence is more readily nurtured. Of course, team members can do this more accurately if they use their colleagues' findings to augment their own assessments.

A comprehensive evaluation developed by an interdisciplinary team can be more effectively conveyed than multiple isolated observations to other interested parties. Families, employers, insurers, and government agencies have various needs for information. Mixed messages can be avoided when expertise is pooled in a team meeting before such information is released.

Interdisciplinary communication can also speed detection of attempts to simulate pathology. Individuals who might be seeking secondary gain may simulate a deficit for a clinician who is perceived as responsible for that problem. Speaking in a faint whisper to a speech therapist may be discounted if projection of a loud voice is reported by other team members. Dramatic swaying in a sinusoidal pattern during formal balance testing is often a marker for simulation. When this is coupled with observation of good balance skills in other settings, the level of suspicion is much higher. Weak hands might be noted to lift heavy bags. Stiff necks occasionally start rotating freely away from clinical settings.

Team members may also share information regarding possible motives for simulation of pathology. Pursuit of legal action or disability claims certainly should not be used to discount the validity of symptoms, since many legitimately injured individuals pursue such claims. Conversely, absence of such activity does not rule out other secondary gain. A family member or significant other may be tied to the patient by the extent of the patient's disability, and recovery might jeopardize the relationship. Attention from therapists may be so highly valued that extra efforts are made to extend treatment.

In other situations, suspicions of malingering can be allayed when team input is requested. Vision or balance problems may legitimately vary with fatigue. Attention to mental tasks may suffer with increased emotional distress. Fluency in a second language may be more severely impaired than in a primary language. Many such factors might appear suspicious at times, but careful review across disciplinary lines can help to weigh the probability of true organic pathology.

These benefits of interdisciplinary teams are generally derived from enhanced communication and cooperation. Regular meetings to discuss cases, as well as program philosophy and strategies, are a logical means of achieving such enhancements. The difficulties involved in finding a time and place to meet may be substantial. The time spent does reduce potential treatment time, and thus revenue is proportionately reduced. This raises the question of whether providers should be allowed greater opportunities to bill such case conferences to insurance carriers and/or patients. When such conferences improve quality of care and increase efficiency of treatment sessions, then the effort and expense are potentially well justified.

Optometry has only recently begun to involve itself substantially in the rehabilitation of brain-injured patients. In spite of institutional barriers discussed earlier, increasing numbers of optometrists have become resources to some of the more established members of the rehabilitation team, particularly for those providing care in outpatient programs. Informal referral patterns have allowed the various practitioners to engage in meaningful clinical collaboration. Perhaps the functional/behavioral approach to the ocular and visual consequences of acquired brain injury has identified these optometrists as kindred souls to members of institutional or private practice rehabilitation programs. These clinical alliances are strengthened by increasing formal recognition in texts on rehabilitation. Thus, classic textbooks used by physiatrists contain chapters on interdisciplinary teams[12] but have not featured information on the potential role of optometrists. However, one recent text showed interest in optometric interventions, particularly vision therapy and optical devices,[8] while another included an entire chapter on rehabilitative optometric interventions in adult acquired brain-injured patients.[13] Nevertheless, until such time as the political and interprofessional issues are resolved, allowing for more privileging of optometrists in rehabilitative hospital units, the profession should strive to make itself and its value in patient care more universally known. This can be accomplished by presentations to in-service programs and grand rounds as well as participation in support groups for patients with acquired brain injury.

References

1. Kraus JF, Sorenson SB. Epidemiology. In: Silver JM, Yudofsky SC, Hales RE, eds. Neuropsychiatry of Traumatic Brain Injury. Washington DC: American Psychiatric Press, 1994:3-41.

2. Torner JC, Schootman M. Epidemiology of closed head injury. In: Rizzo M, Tranel D, eds. Head Injury and Postconcussive Syndrome. New York: Churchill Livingstone, 1995:19-46.

3. Max W, MacKenzie EJ, Rice DP. Head injuries: costs and consequences. J Head Trauma Rehab 1991;6:76.

4. Lewin ICF. The Cost of Disorders of the Brain. Washington D.C.: The National Foundation for the Brain 1992:35.

5. Richter EF. Orthopedic impairments. In: Eisenberg MG, Glueckauf RL, Zaretsky HH, eds. Medical Aspects of Disability. 2nd ed. New York: Springer, 1999:329-41.

6. Bruyere SM, DeMarinis RK. Legislation and rehabilitation service delivery. In: Eisenberg MG, Glueckauf RL, Zaretsky HH, eds. Medical Aspects of Disability. 2nd ed. New York: Springer, 1999:679-95.

7. Strasser DC, Falconer JA. Linking treatment to outcomes through teams. Topics in Stroke Rehabilitation 1997; 4:15-27.

8. Bontke CF, Boake C. Principles of brain injury rehabilitation. In: Braddom RL, ed. Physical Medicine & Rehabilitation. Philadelphia: Saunders, 1996:1027-51.

9. Ludwig BI. Post-traumatic seizures. Physical Medicine and Rehabilitation: State of the Art Reviews 1993;7(3):461-73.

10. Herdman SJ, Helminski JO. Vestibular deficits in the head-injured patient. Physical Medicine and Rehabilitation: State of the Art Reviews 1993;7(3):559-68.

11. Suchoff IB, Kapoor N. The occurance of ocular and visual dysfunction in an acquired brain injured patient sample. J Am Optom Assoc 1999 May;70:301-8.

12. Currie DM, Marburger RA. Writing therapy referrals and treatment plans and the interdisciplinary team. In: Delisa JA, ed. Rehabilitation Medicine. Philadelphia: J. B. Lippincott, 1998:145-57.

13. Suchoff IB, Gianutsos R. Rehabilitative optometric interventions for the adult with acquired brain injury. In: Grabois M, Garrison SJ, Hart KA, Lemkuhl LD, eds. Physical Medicine and Rehabilitation: The Complete Approach. Malden, MA: Blackwell Science, 2000:608-20.

The Neuropsychological Evaluation: A Pathway to Understanding the Sequelae of Brain Injury

Mary R. Hibbard, Ph.D., ABPP
Wayne A. Gordon, Ph.D., ABPP
Barbara Kenner, Ph.D.

Introduction

In medical settings where close relationships between neuropsychologists and optometrists exist, the referral of individuals for assessment and treatment of ocular and visual disturbances following brain injury (BI) is rapidly becoming a standard of clinical practice.[1,2] In addition to the presenting visual disturbances, optometrists receiving these referrals must be cognizant of the range of cognitive and affective challenges that individuals may experience subsequent to BI. Unfortunately, communication between traditional rehabilitation centers and optometric settings is often fragmented, with valuable information obtained from both settings poorly shared for the maximal benefit of the patients served. Although a thorough understanding of the diverse cognitive and affective challenges of patients with BI can be gleaned from neuropsychological evaluations, most optometrists find such reports difficult to interpret. As a result, clinicians' abilities to generalize neuropsychological findings into their clinical approaches to assessment and treatment remain limited.

This chapter provides an overview of a neuropsychological evaluation and descriptions of the most common mechanisms and etiologies of brain injury. The cognitive and affective domains typically assessed in a neuropsychological evaluation are explained, and patterns of behavioral performance following brain injury are highlighted. Modifications of clinical approaches, given identified cognitive and affective deficits for individuals with brain injury and ocular difficulties, are suggested.

Common Mechanisms of Acquired Brain Injury

Acquired brain injuries (ABI) are either traumatic in nature or secondary to medical conditions. These events result in a sudden onset of diverse, and often chronic, physical, cognitive and affective changes for an individual. It is important to consider both etiology and mechanisms of a patient's BI, since these factors will often predict the extent and nature of expected cognitive and affective challenges.

In a traumatic brain injury (TBI), the person experiences a blow to the head of sufficient magnitude to result in either a loss of consciousness or a period of altered mental status. If the duration of loss of consciousness is greater than 20 minutes, the person experiences a "moderate-to-severe" TBI. Approximately 15% of TBIs are considered "moderate-to-severe" with most individuals left with significant changes in physical, cognitive and affective functioning. The remaining 85% of individuals experience a "mild" TBI as defined as a blow to the head followed by an altered mental state or a brief loss of consciousness of less than 20 minutes.[3-4] While the term "mild" reflects the extent of neurological damage, the term in no way reflects the functional consequences of the brain injury on daily activities. Fifteen percent of individuals with mild TBI will exhibit long-term changes in physical, cognitive and affective functioning which may be as severe as those changes observed in individuals with moderate-to-severe TBI.

Three mechanisms of a TBI are possible. In an open head injury, the person experiences a blow to the head in which the skull is penetrated and fractured, e.g., by a bullet penetrating the skull or an object falling on the head and penetrating the skull. Damage following open head injury tends to be localized, with subsequent impairments limited to the areas of the brain damaged by the path of the object entering the head and to the specific location (or the point of impact) within the brain. In a closed head injury, the person experiences a blow to the head that results in direct brain damage at the site of impact as well as less direct brain damage due to inertial forces created within the brain. This type of injury often results in more generalized damage. A closed head injury can result from any event in which the brain is rapidly accelerating within the skull and then comes to an abrupt stop. These inertial forces cause stretching of the brain tissue and bruising of near and distant areas of the brain. Finally, in diffuse axonal injury (for example, in a whiplash event occurring during a car crash), the head is whipped forward and back and from side to side, causing the brain to collide at high velocity with the rough inside surfaces of the skull. This rapid movement causes stretching and tearing of nerve cells (axons) throughout the brain and results in more generalized brain damage.[3-4]

Certain medical conditions can produce an acquired brain injury (ABI) resulting in similar functional difficulties as seen following a TBI. Three conditions can produce brain injury following these medical events: 1) reduced supply of blood or oxygen to the brain, 2) structural damage to the brain, and/or 3) biochemical changes within the brain. Specific adjunct therapies required to treat certain medical conditions (e.g., chemotherapy and radiation) may further compromise long-term functional abilities. While cerebrovascular accidents are the most common acquired brain injury, cerebral aneurysms, arteriovenous malformations, and brain tumors (both malignant and benign) can result in BI. The cognitive and physical impairments following these types of medical events may be localized to the specific area of the brain impacted. Other medical events can also result in BI: anoxia, meningitis/encephalitis, select metabolic events (e.g., poisoning, drug overdose, etc.) and exposure to toxic substances (e.g., mold spores, lead, etc.). These latter medical conditions typically result in more diffuse cognitive and physical consequences.[3-4]

The Neuropsychological Evaluation

A neuropsychological evaluation is an intensive study of the behaviors of a person with suspected or known brain injury.[5] This evaluation involves structured interviews, standardized paper and pencil tests, and select computerized testing to examine current levels of functioning. Since all aspects of behavior can be affected by a brain injury, three aspects of behavior are routinely evaluated within a neuropsychological evaluation: cognitive processes (i.e., how information is processed and remembered), emotions (i.e., how information is moderated by feelings, motivation, and the person's prior experiences), and executive functions (i.e., how information is integrated, managed and expressed). A complete evaluation typically requires six to ten hours of testing, with sessions divided into smaller testing intervals.

Neuropsychological evaluations have the advantage of being objective, safe, portable, and relevant to the functional integrity of the brain. There are two distinguishing characteristics of neuropsychological assessment. These comprise an emphasis on the identification and measurement of psychological deficits and the documentation and description of preserved functions, i.e., the patient's behavioral competencies and strengths.[6] Neuropsychological evaluations provide data and diagnostic formulations that contribute to, or confirm, neurological, medical or psychiatric diagnoses. Neuropsychological findings assume particular diagnostic importance when neurological evaluations, neuroradiological findings (including MRI and CT results) and traditional psychiatric evaluation cannot account for behavioral aberrations that fit a meaningful pattern.[6]

Indications for a Neuropsychological Evaluation

Neuropsychological evaluations are conducted for several purposes: to aid in determining a differential diagnosis; to help with a patient's management, care, rehabilitation or vocational planning; to evaluate the effectiveness of a specific treatment or technique; to provide information in a legal matter; and for research purposes.[6] The primary questions addressed by a neuropsychological evaluation include: What is the nature and extent of impairments? Are the impairments consistent with a brain injury? Are the cognitive impairments permanent? Will there be functional recovery? How will cognitive impairments interfere with daily functioning? What are the service needs of an individual based on his/her profile of deficits and strengths identified in testing?

Neuropsychological assessment is usually deferred until after the acute or postacute phases of recovery from the brain injury. During this early period of recovery, changes in the patient's neuropsychological status can occur so rapidly that information gained one day may be obsolete the next. More often, an initial neuropsychological assessment is completed during the initial three to six months after injury and focuses on short-term treatment goals. Neuropsychological evaluations may be repeated over time to refine treatment interventions, to plan long-term rehabilitation needs, and/or to prepare the individual for vocational or school placement. For individuals with evolving conditions (degenerative diseases, tumors, etc.), neuropsychological evaluations may be serially re-administered to document cognitive stability or decline.

Qualified Examiners

Licensed psychologists trained in both neuropsychology and brain behavior typically complete neuropsychological evaluations. These psychologists usually work in rehabilitation and/or clinical neuropsychological settings (such as a neurological unit or behavioral outpatient setting) where individuals with BI are routinely assessed and treated.

Determination of Neuropsychological Strengths and Deficits

The concept of a behavioral deficit presupposes a prior level of functioning against which the patient's performance may be measured. The level of functioning may be based on normative comparisons, i.e., derived from performances based on an appropriate population of individuals. Population norms are usually age related and sometimes education and gender based. The level of functioning can also be based on individual comparisons, i.e., information derived from the patient's prior history or present characteristics. Such history may be inferred from the amount of schooling received, school records, standardized testing (e.g., Scholastic Achievement Tests), employment records and verbal reports of others. Thus, neuropsychological testing uses both normative and individual comparisons to determine areas of deficit.[5,6]

For cognitively impaired individuals, the least impaired abilities on testing and/or prior social accomplishments are often the best behavioral representatives of a person's pre-injury intellectual abilities and cognitive potential.[7] Typically, a neuropsychological evaluation will include a statement about an individual's estimated "pre-BI" or "pre-morbid" abilities. Such statements are presented along a continuum of cognitive abilities which assumes average intellectual abilities as the median, moving downward to below average, borderline and impaired, and upward to above average, superior and very superior ranges. Discrepancies in performance within and between testing domains are the main approach to defining deficits for an individual, i.e., if a person does well in one area, he/she should do well in other areas of testing. Hence, marked discrepancies in performance for an individual are clear signs of dysfunction.

Test administration within the neuropsychological evaluation is standardized, with an individual's performance on a given test reported as a raw score, a standard score or a percentile. A raw score represents the simple total of correct answers to a given test and, in itself, communicates nothing about the relative value of the patient's performance. Instead, raw scores are typically reported as values of a scale based on the performance of a normative population. As such, each score becomes a statement of its value relative to all scores on that scale. The most widely used metrics are standard scores, i.e., measures of the spread or dispersion of a set of scores around a given mean. Virtually all psychological test data can be converted into standard deviation units for between-test comparisons. Furthermore, scores based on a standard score can be translated into percentiles, another commonly used metric in adult testing. Many psychologists avoid reporting specific scores and instead indicate performance levels in terms of commonly accepted classifications of abilities[8,9] since these terms have general acceptance and relatively clear meanings. These classifications, as noted previously, include in descending order of abilities: very superior, superior, high average, average, low average, borderline and impaired.

Use of Standardized Test Batteries
While standardized test batteries are available, most neuropsychologists prefer to utilize an individualized approach to test selection to best identify cognitive strengths and weaknesses. The scope of cognitive domains assessed in a traditional neuropsychological examination are fairly standard across evaluators and reflect assessment of the known cognitive domains

most likely to be impacted by brain injury. While the specific tests administered will vary among evaluators, the ultimate choice of tests is driven by the information obtained in the initial clinical interview. As the examination progresses, the neuropsychologist continuously tests various hypotheses regarding diagnosis, areas of cognitive strengths and dysfunction, and psychosocial issues which may be contributing to the total behavioral picture. The examiner typically starts with a basic battery that touches on major dimensions of cognitive behaviors, with additional tests selected as the examination proceeds. The patient's strengths and handicaps will also help shape the tests selected.

Assessment of Cognitive Domains

As professionals in vision science are keenly aware, visual abilities are particularly vulnerable to the impact of brain injury. Issues of impaired visual fields, diplopia, intermittent breakdowns in fusional abilities, strabismus, fixation, and pursuit and saccadic eye movements[1,10-14] have been documented within the field of optometry and will therefore not be the primary focus of this chapter. The functional impact of reduced visual perception and visual spatial abilities is a focus of a neuropsychological evaluation since these deficits significantly impact basic academic abilities, i.e., reading, writing, and mathematics, as well as activities of daily living. These deficits contribute to problems in processing speed, memory, attention, sequencing and general motoric functioning. Tests of neglect, visual perception, synthesis, discrimination, spatial orientation and visual-motor coordination are commonly included in a neuropsychological evaluation, and they are utilized to alert the neuropsychologist to the need for optometric referral.[15]

While optometrists are most familiar with psychometric assessment of visual perceptual abilities, neuropsychological assessment includes the evaluation of diverse cognitive and affective abilities that may be impacted by brain injury. These cognitive and affective domains include: intellectual functioning, attention, information processing speed, communication/language skills, memory, executive functioning, mood and behavior.[15-18] A review of these domains and the typical patterns of behaviors noted in individuals following BI are summarized below.

Intellectual Functioning

Intellectual functioning reflects the aggregate of cognitive functioning for the individual at the point of testing. Intellectual functioning assesses both verbal and performance abilities. The impact of the BI on intelligence is often uneven, with some skills impaired and others preserved. The profile of intellectual test performance assists the clinician in establishing hypotheses about impaired functioning and thus guides the selection of additional tests to be used in the remainder of the assessment.[5,6] Verbal abilities are selectively reduced following left brain injury, performance skills are selectively impaired by right hemisphere damage, and more diffuse intellectual impairments are noted following TBI and other diffuse BIs.

Attention

Impaired attention and concentration are common cognitive problems following BI. To understand impairments within this cognitive domain, attention will be divided into auditory, visual and attentional skills.

Auditory attention refers to the ability to attend to information that is presented orally (i.e., information that one hears).

Visual attention refers to the ability to attend to information that is presented visually, including written material, pictures, videos, etc. Visual attention can be broken down into two components: simple and complex. As with auditory attention, visual attention can require either simple or sustained abilities. Individuals with BI are generally able to perform tasks requiring simple visual attention, i.e., the ability to fully attend to or focus on a single visual stimulus. However, most everyday tasks require complex visual attention, i.e., the ability to accurately attend and discriminate between a number of differing competing stimuli presented simultaneously. Individuals with BI may also exhibit decreasing accuracy as tasks become more visually complicated.

Attention span refers to the span, or amount, of new information an individual can attend to the first time it is presented. Individuals with BI may demonstrate a reduction in the amount of information they can attend to.

Sustained attention refers to the ability to maintain involvement in, or focus on, a single activity over a prolonged period of time. Even when the initial span of attention is adequate, individuals with BI may have difficulty filtering out distractions and maintaining concentration on the task at hand.

Divided attention refers to the ability to shift and reshift focus to alternating tasks during the completion of a complex activity (in other words, to perform more than one activity at a time and maintain adequate attention to all aspects of a task). For example, the ability to listen to a verbal presentation, follow written descriptions, and take notes during an interview requires intact divided attention abilities. These abilities are extremely reduced in many individuals with BI.

Information processing speed

Information processing refers to the speed at which information is processed through all the senses, i.e., hearing, vision, taste, touch and smell. Processing speed (e.g., the amount of time required to complete a task) is based on typical performance norms for unimpaired individuals. Following BI, individuals typically experience reduced processing speeds in all sensory modalities. As information becomes more complicated, the individual tends to process information at an even slower pace. In other words, the more complex the information a person needs to process, the longer it will take the person to complete the task. Attempts to rush an individual with reduced processing speed will only result in increased errors in performance and increased frustration.

Response time–Following BI, there is a noticeable slowing in overall response time. As a result, it will take an individual with BI longer to understand, comprehend and respond to information. It will also take such individuals longer to complete simple tasks.

Auditory processing speed–Individuals with BI may take longer to process information that is presented orally. An individual with an auditory processing speed deficit will take a significantly longer time to formulate a response to a question. Thus, these individuals will perform poorly on tasks requiring a rapid verbal response to questions asked in an interview situation.

Visual processing speed–Individuals with BI will take longer to process information that is presented visually. As a result, individuals with brain injury take considerably longer to complete standardized forms than do their peers.

Pacing of information–Pacing refers to the rate at which another individual presents information to a person. Typically, individuals with BI have significant difficulties in keeping abreast of information presented at a normal rate of speed. Typically, these individuals require accommodations, i.e., slowing down the rate at which information is verbally presented to maximize comprehension.

Memory functioning
Memory and learning difficulties are the hallmarks of a brain injury. Common self-reported memory complaints by individuals with BI include poor memory, difficulty learning new information, being forgetful and feeling confused. Family and friends easily can identify these overt cognitive challenges in individuals. As is true within the other cognitive domains, memory abilities are dependent on the relative complexity of the information to be remembered. As task complexity increases, the individual's ability to remember information may decrease. As a result, information is best remembered when presented in a simple, organized, step-by-step manner. Repetition of complex information is typically necessary to ensure ade-

quate learning, storage and long-term retrieval of information. To understand the process of memory and learning in individuals with BI, it is important to understand the way a person encodes, learns and remembers new information.

Encoding–Encoding refers to the individual's ability to acquire and register new incoming information into memory. Due to coexisting difficulties in attention, individuals with BI typically have reduced abilities to encode new information, thus resulting in loss of information over the long term.

Learning–Learning refers to the incremental acquisition of new information. Individuals with BI require an extended number of repetitions to learn new information. Despite additional repetition, their learning abilities continue to be reduced relative to pre-TBI functioning.

Long-term recall–Once new information is encoded, it is stored in memory for ready access at a later point in time. Since persons with BI often are limited in their encoding abilities, the amount of information available for storage and later recall is similarly reduced. Information that is repeated several times to ensure that learning has occurred may be more easily recalled, but reduced relative to pre-BI functioning.

Visual and verbal memory–Information is learned and remembered using both visual and verbal modalities. After a BI, a person may demonstrate greater difficulties in learning and retrieval of information in one modality as opposed to the other. For example, an individual may best remember new information when it is written (visual memory) as contrasted with information that is presented orally (verbal memory). Many individuals with BI require a multimodal (visual and verbal) approach to maximize their memory abilities.

Executive functioning

Executive functioning refers to a variety of skills that interact simultaneously to complete everyday activities effectively. These skills include prioritizing, planning, organizing, flexible thinking, abstraction, problem-solving abilities and the ability to shift rapidly from one task to another. Difficulties in any one of these interactive skills can significantly impact functioning. It is our experience that many individuals with BI exhibit deficits in one or more executive functioning skills. This is nor surprising since executive functioning impairments are hallmarks of frontal lobe injury.[19,20] These deficits have a significant impact on successful vocational, academic and community re-entry.

Prioritization–Prioritizing refers to the ability to arrange tasks in the order they need to be accomplished. Individuals with executive functioning deficits have difficulty deciding the relative ordering of tasks to be completed. When individuals are confronted with several tasks, they may need assistance in prioritizing the activities to complete them in a logical order.

Set shifting abilities–Set shifting refers to the ability to do more than one thing at a time and accomplish all tasks efficiently. In individuals with BI, the ability to shift focus from one task to another is significantly reduced. Attempting to do two tasks simultaneously results in poor performance on both tasks.

Abstract thinking–Abstract thinking refers to the ability to conceptualize and make inferences from information. After a BI, individuals frequently have reduced abilities to think abstractly, typically viewing information in a concrete or factual fashion. For example, individuals with BI may have difficulty explaining how two different items (e.g., an apple and an orange) are alike (i.e., they are both fruits). Their responses will reflect more factual or concrete descriptions of the objects (e.g., they are both round, you can eat them both, etc.).

Planning and organization–Planning and organization involve identifying flexible strategies to complete a task and determining the logical sequence of activities required to achieve this task. These planning and organization skills are significantly reduced in individuals with BI.

Flexible thinking–Flexible thinking refers to the ability to see alternative solutions to an issue or problem, multiple sides of a story, and/or possible consequences of an action. After a BI, individuals often become less flexible in the way they think, tending instead to fixate on one, and only one, interpretation of an issue. When confronted with an unexpected outcome or surprise in their plan, they are unable to draw on alternative solutions or approaches to achieve their goal.

Problem solving–Problem solving refers to the ability to consider alternatives and evaluate which alternative is the most appropriate choice for a situation. Individuals with BI manifest reduced problem-solving skills. Reduced flexibility further limits an individual's ability to generate multiple alternatives to a problem effectively.

Communication impairments
Communication is typically a social, spontaneous and unstructured process. A BI adversely impacts the verbal, nonverbal and pragmatic aspects of communication. While these deficits may be more subtle than the other cognitive difficulties previously discussed, they represent significant challenges following BI.

Organization of verbal responses–Responding to an open-ended question requires the ability to select from a variety of potential responses, prioritize key elements of the presentation, organize the presentation of these facts, and present them in a logical order. These organizational abilities are often challenged in individuals with BI due to underlying deficits in executive functioning, processing speed and memory. As a result, individuals often wander off topic, provide irrelevant details and miss key points of information needed within a typical conversation.

Organization of written responses–Coexisting deficits in organization, prioritization and abstraction negatively impact written discourse for individuals following BI. Typically, individuals with BI have difficulty organizing written content, maintaining topics and/or following external written structure (e.g., outlines).

Maintenance of topic–Inability to organize information either verbally or in writing results in difficulty with topic maintenance. This skill is a critical one for academic achievement and social interactions. Individuals with BI have significant difficulties staying on topic, switching topics during a conversation, and maintaining the "give and take" flow of a normal conversation. Combined, these challenges significantly alter communication abilities.

Understanding figurative/idiomatic language–Understanding figurative/idiomatic language requires an appreciation of the nuances of language, an ability to think abstractly, and to think flexibly. Since these skills may be impaired following BI, individuals often have difficulty understanding jokes or use of sarcasm.

Comprehension of general discussions–Individuals with BI have difficulty comprehending information presented during a conversation, not because of difficulties with understanding what is being said, but because of selective loss of this information due to coexisting memory, attention or information processing deficits.

Word finding abilities–Individuals with BI may display difficulty with finding the specific words they want to use to express themselves, i.e., they may not be able to retrieve names quickly, or they may misname an object or person. These difficulties reflect coexisting memory and organizational deficits that prevent formulation of an effective retrieval strategy.

Self-initiation–Reduced initiation abilities, typically observed as an inability to initiate social conversations, are common difficulties for individuals with BI. These difficulties reflect coexisting difficulties in organization, flexible thinking and rapid information processing speed which are necessary to engage in spontaneous dialogues. As a result, individuals with BI may avoid situations in which they are required to socialize and may be erroneously viewed by others as shy or socially withdrawn.

Eye contact–Individuals with BI may exhibit inappropriate eye contact during conversations. For example, they may avoid eye contact, look everywhere but at the person with whom they are interacting, or stare intently at the other person.

Nonverbal communication–Nonverbal communication refers to the ability to respond to another person through nonverbal approaches, such as nodding one's head, using facial expression or touch to convey concern, etc. Following BI, individuals may exhibit reduced use of nonverbal communication skills.

Use of interpersonal space–Pragmatic change following BI can also result in the inappropriate use of interpersonal space. For example, individuals with BI may stand too close to people or too far away during an interaction.

Affective Challenges after Brain Injury
Given the range of cognitive challenges previously identified, it is of little surprise that individuals with BI experience a range of psychological reactions. Affective reactions can be categorized into three general areas: emotional reactions, difficulties in acceptance of changes in self, and alterations in emotional control.[21]

Emotional reactions
Depression–Depression is the most common emotional reaction following BI.[22] Individuals will exhibit symptoms of sadness, loss of interest in social and physical activities, and feelings of worthlessness and hopelessness. In extreme cases, individuals may present with suicidal ideations. Physical symptoms of depression may also be present and include changes in appetite and weight, loss of energy, and sleep disturbances. Often, depressed individuals will appear withdrawn and may sound emotionally flat.

Anxiety–Individuals often present with signs of generalized anxiety post BI.[22] Anxiety symptoms include nervousness, restlessness and hyperactivity. It is not uncommon for individuals who have experienced a life-threatening event as the precipitator of their BI (e.g., a motor vehicle crash) to exhibit avoidant behaviors and experience nightmares about their injuries.

Accepting changes in self
Perhaps the biggest challenge facing individuals following a BI is learning to accept their "new" self subsequent to the injury and mourn their lost abilities. Psychotherapy and cognitive remediation are often utilized to in-

crease a patient's awareness and appreciation of current cognitive strengths and weaknesses, thereby helping individuals begin to value themselves once again.

Alterations in behavioral control

Behavioral control refers to the ability to evaluate one's internal affect state within a given context or environment and appropriately express or inhibit an overt display of one's emotional reactions depending upon the context or environment. Following BI, a person may have difficulty inhibiting socially inappropriate comments or affective expressions. For example, before the BI, an individual may have been able to keep personal thoughts about a stranger's unusual behaviors to himself; after the BI, the individual may be unable to inhibit expressing these thoughts, thus provoking the stranger by providing unwanted feedback. Similarly, individuals with BI may exhibit extreme emotional reactions in response to minimal provocation. As a result, individuals post BI are often viewed as impulsive, risk taking and unpredictable.

Accommodations Needed when Treating Individuals with BI

Prior to the initial appointment with a patient who has experienced a BI, the optometrist is encouraged to review available neuropsychological reports to obtain a profile of an individual's cognitive and affective strengths and weaknesses. Knowing a person's unique cognitive profile allows the clinician to plan accommodations needed to maximize a clinical assessment and/or treatment session. Table 1 summarizes suggested accommodations for select cognitive and affective domains previously discussed. Use of these accommodations will empower persons with BI to become active members of their treatment team and enhance their abilities to profit from visual rehabilitation efforts.

References

1. Ciuffreda KJ, Suchoff IB, Marrone MA, Ahmann E. Oculomotor rehabilitation in traumatic brain injured patients. J Behav Optom 1996;7(2):31-8.

2. Suchoff IB, Kapoor N, Waxman R, Ference W. The occurrence of ocular and visual dysfunctions in an acquired brain-injured patient sample. J Am Optom Assoc 1999; 70(5):301-08.

3. Dombovy ML. Traumatic brain injury. In: Lazar RB, ed. Principles of Neurologic Rehabilitation. New York: McGraw-Hill Health Professions Division, 1997:79-103.

4. National Institutes of Health. Report of the Consensus Development Conference on the Rehabilitation of Persons with Traumatic Brain Injury. Bethesda, MD: National Institute of Health, 1999.

5. Pliskin NH, Ferman TJ, Lacy M, Wood KC. Neuropsychological assessment. In: Lazar RB, ed. Principles of Neurologic Rehabilitation. New York: McGraw-Hill Health Professions Division, 1997:579-88.

6. Lezak MD. Neuropsychological Assessment. 3rd ed. New York: Oxford Press, 1995.

7. Jastak JF. A rigorous criterion of feeble-mindedness. J Abnorm Soc Psychol 1949;44:367-78.

8. Matarazzo JD. Wechsler's Measurement and Appraisal of Adult Intelligence. 5th ed. Baltimore: Williams and Wilkins, 1972.

9. Wechsler D. Weschsler Adult Intelligence Scale. Rev. New York: The Psychological Corporation, 1981.

10. Baker RS, Epstein A. Ocular motor abnormalities from head trauma. Surv Opthalmol 1991;35(4):245-67.

11. Trobe HL, Lorber ML, Schlezinger NS. Isolated homonymous hemianopia. Arch Ophthalmol 1973; 89:377-81.

12. Gianutsos R, Ramsey G, Perlin R. Rehabilitative optometric services for survivors of acquired brain injury. Arch Phys Med Rehabil 1988; 69:573-8.

13. Liu D. Post-traumatic visual disorders: Part II. Management and rehabilitation. In: Stone LR, ed. Physical Medicine and Rehabilitation; Neurologic and Orthopedic Sequelea of Traumatic Brain Injury. Philadelphia: Hanley and Belfus, Inc, 1989.

14. Schlageter K, Gray K, Shaw R et al. Incidence and treatment of visual dysfunctions in traumatic brain injury. Brain Inj 1993;7:439-48.

15. Adams RL, Parsons OA, Culbertson JL, Nixon SJ, eds. Neuropsychology for Clinical Practice: Etiology, Assessment and Treatment of Common Neurological Disorders. Washington, DC: American Psychological Association, 1996.

16. Parker RS. Traumatic Brain Injury and Neuropsychological Impairment: Sensoriomotor, Cognitive, Emotional and Adaptive Problems of Children and Adults. New York: Springer-Verlag, 1990.

17. Walsh K. Neuropsychology: A Clinical Approach. 3rd ed. New York: Churchill-Livingstone, 1994.

18. Stringer AY. Adult Neuropsychological Diagnosis. Philadelphia: F. A. Davis Company, 1995.

19. Damasio AR, Anderson SW. The frontal lobes. In: Heilman KM, Valenstein E, eds. Clinical Neuropsychology. New York: Oxford Press, 1993:409-60.

20. Mateer CA. Rehabilitation of individuals with frontal lobe impairments. In: Leon-Carrion J, ed. Neuropsychological Rehabilitation: Fundamentals, Innovations and Directions. Delray Beach, FL: GR/St. Lucie Press, 1997:285-300.

21. Machuca F, Carrasco JM, Gonzalez AM, Rodrigues-Durate R, Leon-Carrion J. Training for social skills after brain injury. In: Leon-Carrion J, ed. Neuropsychological Rehabilitation: Fundamentals, Innovations and Directions. Delray Beach, FL: GR/St. Lucie Press, 1997:453-82.

22. Hibbard MR, Uysal S, Kepler K et al. Axis I psychopathology in individuals with traumatic brain injury. Head Trauma Rehabil 1998;13:24-39.

Table 1.
Accommodations for Cognitive and Affective Deficits in Individuals with BI

Cognitive Deficits Identified	Suggested Accommodations
Attention Deficits	Work only on one task at a time in session Limit auditory and visual distractions within testing room Provide scheduled breaks within planned treatment sessions Make sessions as interactive as possible to enhance patient's attention Redirect the patient when he/she becomes distracted
Reduced Information Processing Speed	Speak slowly, stopping frequently to check comprehension Avoid speaking in a loud voice. Use a normal tone of voice Do not attempt to rush the patient with a task Allow additional time for the patient to formulate responses to questions Encourage family members to assist the patient with (or provide assistance with) completion of written forms
Memory Impairments	Repeat information several times to ensure comprehension Check the patient's understanding of new information by asking him/her to restate the information in his/her own terms Do not assume a patient will remember new information between sessions. Inconsistency is the hallmark of BI Provide written documentation whenever possible to augment verbal discussions Present new information in small, concise chunks to maximize learning Ask structured questions, as opposed to open-ended questions Encourage the patient to write down instructions, home assignments, etc., for later review
Executive Functioning Deficits	Keep unexpected events to a minimum Provide information in a factual manner, avoiding use of abstract concepts whenever possible Prepare patient in advance when session focus will be shifting Provide alternative solutions to a problem and empower the patient to select the best choice Provide a written agenda of things to be accomplished in session Provide a written outline which summarizes specific steps to be followed for completion of a home therapy program

Cognitive Deficits Identified	Suggested Accommodations
Communication Deficits	Limit the use of open-ended questions during verbal questioning and on written forms Use structured questions (yes/no format; multiple choice) whenever possible Redirect the patient when he/she wanders "off topic" in discussions Cue patients who experience word-finding difficulties Encourage appropriate eye contact and use of interpersonal space Model use of nonverbal gestures when appropriate
Affective Changes	A flat affect should not be interpreted as a sign of lack of interest Reassurance, education and structure are useful techniques to minimize anxiety for a patient Encourage realistic assessment of the patient's current abilities Avoid focusing only on the patient's deficits Provide neutral, but directed, feedback when the patient behaves inappropriately Suggest brief breaks whenever the patient becomes irritable or agitated Offer alternative activities when a patient begins to show signs of agitation

Neuropsychological Consequences of Mild Brain Injury and Optometric Implications

Rosamond Gianutsos, Ph.D.
Irwin B. Suchoff, O.D., D.O.S.

Mild traumatic brain injury (MTBI) has been defined by a panel of specialists convened under the auspices of the American Congress of Rehabilitation Medicine.[1] The diagnostic criteria for MTBI are tabulated in Table 1.

Thus, MTBI includes situations where the head has been struck, the head has struck an object, or the brain has undergone acceleration/deceleration (i.e., whiplash) without direct external trauma to the head. Conversely, MTBI excludes other forms of acquired brain injury such as stroke, anoxia, tumor, encephalitis and dementia.

The consensus on diagnostic criteria is not paralleled with respect to terminology. Many use the term postconcussion syndrome. Especially among individuals whose symptoms have not resolved within a few months, there is a concern that "mild" minimizes the impact of this condition. Not long ago a spirited discussion in the Traumatic Brain Injury Support Group (TBI-SPRT) addressed several substitutes for mild, including: minor, minimal, subtle, and ambiguous. (TBI-SPRT is accessible on the Internet at www.sasquatch.com/tbi/subscribe.com) We prefer the concept of subtle brain injury. However, for the remainder of this chapter the much maligned, but recognized, term mild brain injury (MBI) will be used.

Table 1. Diagnostic Criteria for Mild Traumatic Brain Injury Include at Least One of the Following:

- any period of loss of consciousness
- any loss of memory for events immediately before or after the accident
- any alteration in mental state at the time of the accident (e.g., feeling dazed, disoriented or confused)
- focal neurological deficit(s) that may or may not be transient, but where the severity of the injury does not exceed the following loss of consciousness of approximately 30 minutes or less
- after 30 minutes, an initial Glasgow Coma Scale (GCS) of 13-15
- post-traumatic amnesia (PTA) not greater than 24 hours

The most important neuropsychological finding regarding MBI is that symptoms resolve within three months in the vast majority of cases.[2] In the short run, probably the best course for the rehabilitative clinician is to maintain a positive outlook and to encourage the individual to seek further treatment if symptoms persist beyond three months. One must avoid statements which, though intended to be supportive, may encourage symptoms to persist. This concept was expressed by the author Marcel Proust, cited by Putnam and Millis:[3] "For each ailment that doctors cure with medications they produce 10 others in healthy individuals by inoculating them with that pathogenic agent a thousand times more virulent than all the microbes - the idea that they are ill."

However, without setting up an expectancy that symptoms will persist, the clinician should offer counseling regarding the types of situations or conditions that could trigger the need for further treatment: for example, difficulties in school- or work-related performance or in activities requiring sustained concentration, management of behavioral consequences such as increased irritability, and anhedonia.

The clinical challenge is with those MBI survivors who have persisting symptoms. Cicerone and Kalmar[2] correctly point out that there are undoubtedly several underlying postconcussion syndromes including cognitive, affective, somatic and sensory domains; these are listed in Table 2. It should be noted that symptoms typical of MBI, as previously cited and summarized in Table 1, clearly reflect these different domains. Patients report symptoms from some, but rarely all, of these domains.

Table 2. Symptoms Typical of MBI (when not accounted for by other causes)

Physical—nausea, vomiting, dizziness, headache, blurred vision, sleep disturbance, quickness to fatigue, lethargy, or other sensory loss

Cognitive—deficits in attention, concentration, perception, memory, speech/language, executive functions

Behavioral—changes in the degree of emotional responsivity, e.g, irritability, quickness to anger, disinhibition, or emotional lability

Persistent MBI features a discordance between subjective and objective symptoms. In some situations subjective symptoms exceed objective ones. How many of the above symptoms have we all experienced at one time or another? It is not uncommon for patients to be quite verbal in their subjective complaints, to a degree that seems inconsistent with the specific complaint, e.g., a detailed exposition about how they forgot something three months ago. Not infrequently, there is some form of litigation, suggesting other motivational issues. The challenge for the clinician is to maintain a neutral posture and to seek objective indicators, bearing in mind that in most cases the subjective symptoms have a basis in fact.

Some years ago, following a fall at work, one gentleman's symptoms were so ambiguous that he was not even evaluated for brain injury for a year. Although his brain scans were negative, cognitive testing and subjective symptoms suggested MBI. Optometric evaluation showed binocular and perceptual problems and the patient received a long course of optometric vision therapy as well as neuropsychological (cognitive) rehabilitation. He had a positive but incomplete response to treatment. Meanwhile, the validity of his symptomatology and complaints was challenged by independent medical evaluations, with the implication that his problems were basically psychiatric. Seven years later, when his lawsuit came to trial, he had a new set of scans, including the newly available and more sensitive MRI. The more sensitive tests revealed unambiguous evidence of brain injury. However, the absence of "hard" evidence of central nervous system damage or dysfunction is often not sufficient to rule out brain injury, even with present technology.

Some conditions are by their nature more evident subjectively than objectively. For example, word-finding problems are often reported by seemingly articulate patients. Occasionally, one may observe some halting speech, but rarely do such problems show up on formal testing. Here the problem may be a lack of sensitive testing instruments. Only recently have some tests of word finding appeared which incorporate precise reaction time measures. It is also likely that we do not observe breakdowns in word finding because most patients come up with an acceptable synonym and the problem passes unnoticed by the outside observer.

The neuropsychologist needs to evaluate carefully the individual's pre-injury level of functioning and personality style. At greatest risk are people who had achieved much and held themselves to a high standard and who are intolerant of cognitive failures. Thomas Kay, a neuropsychologist who has written several insightful articles on MBI, [4,5] describes this syndrome as a "shaken sense of self" with "loss of confidence in their own ability both to perform as they used to in cognitively challenging situations and to be able to predict or anticipate their own performance in any given situation."[6] For such individuals, even a relatively small chink in the armor is devastating.

Another case illustrates recovery from persistent MBI in which optometric intervention was particularly helpful. This individual is a tenured professor who sustained multiple trauma as a pedestrian hit by a car. Although he only had one acute seizure, he was placed on prophylactic anticonvulsant medication. He experienced diplopia, which significantly interfered with activities such as reading. Optometric evaluation revealed a strabismus, which was successfully treated with prisms and vision therapy. Neuropsychological evaluation showed information processing inefficiency, including problems with attention, concentration and the formation of new memory. He had difficulty in problem solving; although he was often creative in constructing alternative hypotheses, he would, at times, miss the obvious. He reported needing excessive sleep—a problem which was totally foreign to him. Neuropsychological rehabilitation addressed the cognitive problems by offering techniques and counseling regarding ways he could manage or compensate for his deficits. The need for sleep resolved when the neurologist discontinued the antiseizure medication. He also began to resume aspects of his professional work, e.g., editorial reviews, working on manuscripts begun prior to his injury, following up on ongoing research projects, becoming embroiled in departmental politics.

Nearly a year after his injury he returned to his full-time position. He completed his first semester with little difficulty evident to others. However, he was advised to keep a log of his difficulties in his computerized personal information manager. His observations reveal much of how MBI interferes with the activities of daily living of a professional person; they are paraphrased in Table 3.

In some cases it is difficult to keep treatment from becoming protracted. There comes a time when the clinician may have to bring the active treatment phase to a close and to encourage the individual to get on with life, such as is possible. While the professor did not remain in therapy longer than necessary, he did need some help coming to terms with the likelihood that some problems would continue and that he would have to expend much effort in compensation, at least for the foreseeable future.

The decision when to discontinue efforts to resolve the residual symptoms is best conceived as a transition from restoration to compensation as a therapy goal. People differ in how ready they are to make this shift. The therapist can help by playing down the notion of "giving up" or "accepting" one's deficits. A more positive image of the self as manager should be encouraged. The manager sets priorities and decides which mountains to scale, which to defer, and which to go around. Further, an emphasis in treatment on those things the person can do well should be followed up with efforts to find life situations in which those capabilities are used and the residual deficits are not needed.

It is important to mention another possible scenario, albeit less common. This is the situation where objectively-based symptoms exceed the subjec-

> **Table 3. Professor's Log of Difficulties upon Return to Work Life**
>
> - Experiences seem often new if I haven't done them for a month or two, e.g., friends I don't recall (names and faces). Not entirely unpleasant, but distressing. Seems to be especially a problem with people I've met the past year or two, less with friends of longer standing
> - Don't know people's names when I meet them in the hall; in meetings which meet several times I can't identify people or names
> - Writing proposal ... could not remember previous one, can't remember what we measured or found
> - Found a paper and proposal I had written just before the accident; have no recollection of having written them. They sound OK, but it's like reading someone else's work. I have to think about what's said and to try to understand it
> - A few hours after I told real estate agent about a co-op, forgot that I had discussed it with him; didn't remember telling W about the notebook computer; couldn't recall I had returned call from X: he called Saturday, I returned the call Sunday, by Monday I had forgotten and called him again
> - Couldn't remember a confrontational conversation I'd had with Y a few months ago. After he mentioned it I could only vaguely recall where it happened, but nothing about what was said
> - Forgot to send atty. letter and release; forgot committee meetings; forgot appointment with the Dean; forgot teaching presentation; forgot to grade student papers and to bring next essay assignment
> - Could not remember simple traffic instructions
> - Couldn't figure out how to get possessives, e.g., earth's: apostrophe or not?; couldn't spell diligence, useful, repetitious, concentrate, mystic
> - Hard to concentrate on things, e.g., review of Z's paper, kept forgetting and getting distracted. Left it for four days and forgot most of what I had thought about it

tive ones. When there are other injuries, symptoms of MBI may be obscured. For example, in instances where there is spinal cord injury along with MBI, the consequences of the latter may not be fully recognized by the patient. Some rehabilitation professionals consider this an occult brain injury. Also, some neuropsychological impairment may not be evident until the individual returns to the challenges of work or school.

Optometric Implications

Optometrists are sometimes the first health care professional to encounter the patient who has an undiagnosed MBI. The very nature of the "shaken sense of self" and the inability to conduct activities of daily living as before leads some of these patients or their agents to conclude that "something is wrong with my eyes." Consequently, during the history interview all patients should be questioned whether there was a recent or previous incident that involved injury to the head. With adults, this can bring the patient back to an auto or sports accident that occurred months or even years before. The follow-up question then is whether the patient noted a change in his/her life following the incident. We know of instances where the response is something of the nature of.... "you know, I felt I became another person," or.... "yes, that was the time I began having a lot of arguments with my spouse (and/or) my children." If this is the case, referral to a physiatrist and/or a neuropsychologist is in order to confirm or deny the diagnosis of MBI.

This same line of questioning is particularly important for children who have been referred to the optometrist because of a learning disability or an attention deficit disorder. Again, the parent might well recall a playground incident where the child sustained a blow to the head by a swing, or a fall on a concrete surface; the parent will frequently become aware of changes in the child's behavior coincident with the injury. It has been our experience that if the diagnosis of MBI is subsequently made, the educational strategy and management of the child improves as a result of understanding the child as the victim of an accident rather than simply attaching a label to him or her.

We offer the following "clinical pearls" to use once it has been determined that the patient has incurred MBI.

1. Schedule the patient for more time per visit than your usual policy. It is particularly important that you give these patients time to express themselves and provide yourself enough time to truly listen. Many of these patients have not had this type of treatment. To all outward appearances they appear "normal," so some other health care practitioners have concluded that there is an underlying neurosis and have casually dismissed the patient's complaints. Conducting the history as a two-way conversation fosters trust, which we have found to be a key element in the treatment strategy and successful clinical outcome.

2. Perform a complete primary care eye and vision evaluation and be attuned to conditions and management issues that are important considerations with MBI patients. We have reported on the prevalence of dry eye, photosensitivity and the need for careful refraction and clinical thinking regarding the type of lens to be prescribed for the population of acquired brain-injured (ABI) patients.[7] These considerations also apply to the MBI subgroup. We have found that these patients are also prone to subtle visual field defects that require more functionally-based testing than is possible with modern static or kinetic methods.[8] Finally, our experience concurs with the research of Hellerstein et al.[9] They documented a statistically significant higher prevalence of impaired convergence-related functions, pursuit eye movements, and symptomatology in their experimental group of MBI patients than in their age-matched nonMBI group.

3. Be aware that a number of pharmaceutical agents that are prescribed for these patients might have adverse effects on the physical and functional aspects of the visual system. These include antiseizure, antidepressant and some analgesic agents. Sometimes medications with fewer side effects can be substituted, or the medications withdrawn. This of course requires consultation with the attending neurologist or physiatrist. However, if the medication or dosage cannot be changed, the optometrist must take the side effects into account. For example, progressive addition lenses might be considered for prepresbyopic individuals whose medical status and pharmaceutical management result in variation of accommodative ability.

4. Finally, remember that the patient with MBI presents particular challenges. It is certainly true that some of these individuals cannot return to their former occupations and social roles for months, or even years. Impaired functioning and symptoms, such as a marred ability to concentrate, intermittent vertigo, or sleep disorders leads to the "shaken sense of self," which in turn can lead to anxiety, depression or other social and psychological problems.[10] However, it must be kept in mind that in the majority, a return to much if not all of the patient's former life is the case. Consequently, the optometrist must, as was discussed earlier in this article, seek to understand and provide care that ameliorates the visual consequences of MBI, but at the same time be careful to not reinforce or exacerbate the patient's sense of illness.

References

1. American Congress of Rehabilitation Medicine. Mild Traumatic Brain Injury of the Head Injury Interdisciplinary Special Interest Group. Definition of mild traumatic brain injury. J Head Trauma Rehab 1993; 8:86-7.

2. Cicerone KD, Kalmar K. Persistent postconcussion syndrome: the structure of subjective complaints after mild traumatic brain injury. J Head Trauma Rehab 1995;10:1-17.

3. Putnam S, Millis SR. Psychosocial factors in the development and maintenance of chronic somatic and functional symptoms following mild traumatic brain injury. Advances Med Psychotherapy 1994;7:1-22.

4. Kay T. Minor head injury: an introduction for professionals. Washington, DC: National Head Injury Foundation, 1986.

5 Kay T, Newman B, Cavallo M, Ezrachi O, Resnick M. Toward a neuropsychological model of functional disability after mild traumatic brain injury. Neuropsychol 1992;6:371-84.

6. Kay T. Neuropsychological diagnosis: disentangling the multiple determinants of functional disability after mild traumatic brain injury. Phys Med Rehab: State of the Art Reviews; 6:109-27.

7. Suchoff IB, Gianutsos R, Ciuffreda KJ, Groffman S. Vision impairment related to acquired brain injury. In: Silverstone B, Lang MA, Rosenthal B, Faye EE, eds. The Lighthouse Handbook on Vision Impairment and Rehabilitation. New York: Oxford University Press, 2000:241-61.

8. Gianutsos R, Suchoff IB. Visual fields after brain injury. In: Scheiman M, ed. Understanding and Managing Vision Deficits—A Guide for Occupational Therapists. Thorofare, NJ: Slack, 1997:333-58.

9. Hellerstein LF, Freed S, Maples WC. Vision profile of patients with mild brain injury. J Am Optom Assoc 1995;66:634-39.

10. Marion DDW. Pathophysiology and initial neurosurgical care: future directions. In:Horn LJ, Zasler ND, eds. Medical Rehabilitation of Traumatic Brain Injury. Philadelphia: Hanley & Belfus, 1996:29-52.

Reprinted with permission from the Journal of Behavioral Optometry 1998;9(1):3-6.

Accommodation in Acquired Brain Injury

Stephen Leslie, B Optom

Introduction

Accommodation is very commonly affected by acquired brain injury (ABI), especially traumatic brain injury (TBI). Not uncommonly, there is also an associated convergence dysfunction, either due to primary effects on convergence function or as a secondary consequence of severe accommodative dysfunction. Stroke (CVA) less commonly results in accommodative dysfunction due to its more discrete and localized nature. Nevertheless, the location of a stroke is significant, since vascular damage to the brainstem is likely to have much more significant effects on accommodation, convergence and oculomotor cranial nerve function than in most other regions of the brain.

The degree of accommodative dysfunction subsequent to ABI can range from mild to severe, but the effects on activities of daily living may be dramatic. Accommodative dysfunction can prevent the person from returning to work, severely limit ability to read or use a computer, and limit the progress of other rehabilitative services involving near visual tasks.

The neuro-ophthalmological literature generally only mentions the high incidence of accommodative-convergence sequelae of closed head injuries without significant differential diagnosis or options for management. The general impression of the available literature is that such dysfunctions may improve with time in only a minority of cases. However, while many accommodative-convergence dysfunctions in ABI do not improve spontaneously over time, it is frequently possible to manage the effects, and in some cases eliminate the dysfunction, simply with lenses and optometric vision therapy. This often results in dramatic improvements in visual function in work, study, and other activities of daily living, with commensurate improvements in quality of life.

At the same time, knowledge of the presence and practical effects of an accommodative dysfunction in a patient with ABI can frequently help other rehabilitative professionals to adjust their programs accordingly. Treatment of the visual dysfunction can often remove a significant visual barrier to rehabilitative progress. For example, in occupational therapy and speech therapy, near visual activities, especially computers, are an integral part of rehabilitation.

The traditional view of accommodative function holds that it is primarily initiated by response to blur.[1-3] However, current theory holds that there is a learned component determined by proximal information about the target.[4-6] The infant learns to accommodate by grasping near objects, with the kinesthetic feedback providing proximal information to the visual system to facilitate accurate accommodation.

It is helpful to conceptualize accommodation dysfunctions in ABI as a disturbance or loss of learned ability to change accommodation in visual space appropriately. This spatial concept of accommodation provides a practical way to understand dysfunctions of accommodative skills, such as accuracy, facility and sustenance. It also suggests an effective model for the use of lenses and vision therapy for ABI patients to help them relearn control of their disrupted accommodative system.

It is easy to assume that some areas of the brain involved with accommodation have been damaged beyond repair by a CVA or the local and global effects of TBI. However, while accommodative function frequently does not recover completely, the degree of spontaneous recovery in some patients, and the significant changes in performance as a result of lens application and vision therapy in other patients, strongly suggests the possibility of successful rehabilitation of accommodation for many people with ABI.

While admitting the limited repair mechanisms of the brain, Zost[7] contends that mechanisms of neuroplasticity may aid recovery from cerebral injury. One mechanism, unmasking and reprogramming of neural pathways, essentially enables other pathways, through repeated use, to assume the function of damaged neurons. This only occurs where the demand for function is high, and the brain may still not recover full function. Nevertheless, there is potential for the brain to relearn visual functions through practice, such as with optometric vision therapy.

Peachey has proposed a minimum attention model for efficient vision function. This essentially conceptualizes accommodative-convergence function as a learned (and later automatic) visual skill that operates without significant conscious effort or cognitive attention. Thus, the higher order processing and association of visual information occurs easily and for extended periods.[8] However, when a person with ABI requires conscious effort to clear blurred images, such as when reading, the attention involved diverts cognitive resources from information processing and retention, resulting in reduced concentration and comprehension. Remediation of accommodative dysfunction in ABI must involve the redevelopment of normal accommodative ability which, with practice, can operate with minimal attention again. Essentially, a previously automatic system of focus, caused to be a conscious process by ABI, should be helped by lenses and vision therapy to regain automatic function. Howell has developed a revised classification of accommodation-convergence disorders which is relevant to the effects of ABI on accommodation.[9]

The discussion below of accommodative dysfunction in ABI will relate primarily to TBI and CVA, but the principles and practice apply equally to other neurological conditions which may have effects on accommodative function. These include multiple sclerosis, myasthenia gravis (where accommodative dysfunction may be the first sign of the condition), myotonic dystrophy, Wilson's disease, encephalitis and meningitis, decompression sickness and Parkinsonism. This chapter will review the frequency and possible diagnoses of accommodative dysfunctions as a consequence of ABI, including accommodative insufficiency and fatigue, accommodative excess, and accommodative infacility and inertia. I will also describe what I consider the most valid and practical procedures for assessment of accommodative insufficiency and fatigue, infacility, inertia and excess. In many cases of mild to moderate TBI or CVA, the patient is able to verbalize accurate indications of symptoms, as well as responses to tests of accommodative function. However, in many cases patients may have verbal or cognitive deficits which limit the reliability of subjective history and testing. If subjective assessment is not possible or reliable, objective assessment procedures must be used to obtain valid measures of accommodative function to determine if accommodation is affecting the patient's ability to enjoy activities of daily life (ADLs), as well as to benefit maximally from visual and other rehabilitative services. People with ABI frequently demonstrate specific syndromes of accommodative dysfunctions. These will also be discussed.

Prevalence of Accommodative Dysfunctions in ABI

Gianutsos et al.[10] found that 18 of 26 patients with head injury had accommodative insufficiency. Accommodative problems were often interactive with other visual problems. The amplitude of accommodation was often approximately two diopters below age-expected, which they attributed to overall weakness as well as focal lesions.

Kowal[11] found 36% of 161 head-injured patients demonstrated one or more acquired accommodative problems, with about half recovering within 12 months after injury. Poor accommodation was diagnosed if the subject under 35 years of age complained of near blur that was improved by lenses and usually confirmed by formal measurement of positive relative accommodation and/or nearpoint of accommodation. He diagnosed pseudomyopia if the patient had subjectively blurred vision for distance that was improved with a myopic correction, no history of previous myopia, and when the cycloplegic refraction indicated emmetropia or low hyperopia (nearly all cases) or far less myopia. The adequacy of cycloplegia was assessed by the lack of increase of myopia for near retinoscopy versus distance retinoscopy. He found that nine patients had poor accommodation and convergence insufficiency, seven had convergence insufficiency and pseudomyopia, and four had deficient accommodation. However, these diagnoses must be considered in relation to the categories of accommodative excess and spasm of the near reflex.

Al-Qurainy[12] reported that approximately 20% of patients with midfacial trauma had an accommodative dysfunction. Harrison[13] reported a case of a 20-year-old male who suffered a head injury in an automobile accident and who still had a large difference in amplitudes of accommodation between the two eyes three years later. Roca[14] reported 5 of 15 patients with whiplash who had reduced accommodation and prism vergences.

Ohtsuka et al.[15] diagnosed accommodative insufficiency and slow accommodative responses in a patient complaining of blurred and double near vision subsequent to a middle cerebral artery embolism. In Ohtsuka's case, there was no apparent involvement of the midbrain or oculomotor nerves, yet accommodation was significantly affected. However, the complex neurological control of accommodation makes it very vulnerable to ABI.

The Neurology of Accommodation

The ciliary muscle, which produces accommodative lens changes, is innervated by the autonomic nervous system with input from both the sympathetic[16] and parasympathetic components.[17]

The afferent impulses reach the visual cortex via the optic nerve, optic chiasm, optic tract, lateral geniculate body and optic radiations.[18] The efferent pathway of the sympathetic system involves the cervical sympathetic trunk, superior cervical ganglion and the trunk of the internal carotid to the cavernous plexus; it enters the eye via the long ciliary nerves and short ciliary nerves via the ciliary ganglion.[13]

The parasympathetic innervation pathway to accommodation involves the visual cortex, hypothalamus and Edinger-Westphal nucleus. It then travels from the midbrain via the third cranial nerve to the ciliary ganglion and enters the eye through the short ciliary nerves.

As a result of the complex distribution of the dual innervations to accommodation, many TBIs are likely to affect the innervation and function of accommodation due to the pervasive effects of brain swelling and hemorrhages. CVA is less likely to impair accommodative function due to the frequent focal nature of the cerebrovascular lesion, although the location and severity of the hemorrhage or infarct will determine if accommodation is impaired. Further, the balance of dual autonomic system innervation to accommodation can be affected by general system changes, as well as by medications used to control sequelae such as hypertension, diabetes, depression and epilepsy.

Symptoms of Accommodative Dysfunction

The symptoms of accommodative dysfunction are most noticeable in association with near visual tasks, but can also occur in many other activities of daily living, such as slowness in changing focus from dashboard instruments to the road while driving. Symptoms typically reported by people who have an accommodative problem as a result of an ABI include:

- intermittent blurred vision at distance, near, or both distances
- visual problems more severe later in the day or when fatigued
- problems focusing on near tasks, or changing focus from near to far, or far to near
- headaches, typically frontal or temporal, but less frequently occipital
- pain around the eyes during visual activities
- lid squinting
- closing one eye when reading or engaged in other concentrated visual activities
- reading problems, such as difficulty concentrating and having to reread for comprehension
- words appearing to move or run together when reading
- losing place and missing words when reading
- ocular discomfort

While reduced concentration and comprehension are commonly associated with accommodative dysfunctions in the nonABI population, the effect on comprehension in a patient with ABI may be much more deleterious. In my experience, the attention necessary to compensate after ABI for fatiguing and inaccurate accommodation when attempting to read frequently results in dramatically reduced information processing and rapid loss of reading concentration. Management of the accommodative dysfunction may produce a disproportionate improvement in reading concentration, comprehension, and processing deficits which otherwise may have been attributed

Table 1. Assessment of Accommodation and Expected Minimum Accommodative Performance			
Parameter of Accommodation	Usual Method	When Usual Method Not Feasible (ABI)	Expected Minimum Performance
Accuracy	Cross cylinder	Near retinoscopy	Lag of +0.25 to +0.75D
Amplitude	Pushup Pushdown (pullaway)	Near retinoscopy	Minimum amplitude for age
Stability	Often not determined	Near retinoscopy	Consistent lag when reading
Flexibility/inertia	Flippers	Near retinoscopy with flippers	9-10 cycles per minute +/-2.00D; response <1 second

to significant cognitive deficits. I have also seen cases where performance on neuropsychological testing improves dramatically when previously unrecognized accommodative dysfunctions are appropriately managed.

Clinical Assessment of Accommodative Parameters
General comments
It is important to assess all facets of accommodation clinically.[19] When only one aspect of accommodation (e.g., amplitude) is assessed, it is possible that other accommodative dysfunctions are missed. It is also useful to measure positive relative accommodation (PRA, minus to blur), negative relative accommodation (NRA, plus to blur), and the accommodative convergence to accommodation ratio (AC/A). Addition of plus lenses to best visual acuity is a simple way of measuring the necessary lens for best near visual function, but it reveals little of the nature of the accommodative problem.

The parameters of accommodation and methods of assessment for ABI patients are shown in Table 1 and discussed in the following section.

Accommodative accuracy (lag, lead)
Accommodation is expected to lag behind the plane of regard at 40 cm by between +0.25 and +0.75 diopter[20-22] and should be consistent with the near phoria; normal and equal lags of accommodation of the two eyes, combined with low near exophoria, indicate the accommodation and convergence systems are in synchrony and are optimal for the near visual demand. The lag reflects the accuracy of the accommodative response.

Traditional measures of this accommodative measure have used the fused or unfused cross-cylinder test result,[23] but this subjective test has significant sources of inaccuracy.[24,25] Lag or lead of accommodation can be objectively and accurately measured by near/dynamic[22] or Monocular Estimate Method retinoscopy (MEM). This latter method has been shown to be a valid and reliable[26-28] measure of accommodation in response to the target distance stimulus demand, correlating well with an infrared optometer. A strong correlation between the low neutral dynamic retinoscopy value and MEM, as well as the binocular cross-cylinder measurement, has also been demonstrated.[29] In my experience, MEM retinoscopy is a more valid test of accommodative function in free space; it is often the only feasible test when a patient with ABI cannot respond to standardized testing, due to cognitive or verbal factors. When there is a significant difference in lag of accommodation between the two eyes, it suggests the possibility of uniocular trauma or inflammation, an ABI affecting accommodative performance of both eyes unequally, and/or an uncorrected refractive condition.

Accommodative amplitude

Accommodative amplitude is the maximum amount of accommodation that can be used to focus at near. Traditionally the expected minimum amplitude by age is given by the Hofstetter formula:[30-32]

Minimum amplitude of accommodation (diopters) = 15 - (0.25 x age in years)

Thus a decrease in total amount of accommodation will manifest as deficient accommodation and usually lead to accommodative insufficiency, fatigue, and an inability to sustain accommodation for a prolonged period. An absence of accommodative ability (paralysis of accommodation, absolute presbyopia) will naturally present as consistently blurred vision, with no measurable amplitude.

Accommodative amplitude is traditionally measured by the subjective pushup method. A target of appropriate small print is slowly advanced toward one eye, with the other eye occluded. The amplitude is the dioptric equivalent of the distance at which the patient reports the first slightly sustained blur with full effort. In children and some adults, it is advisable to check the pushup amplitude result by the pullaway (pulldown) method, where the target is placed slightly closer to the patient than the pushup blur point and pulled away until it is read or reported as clear.[33] It can also be measured by the minus lens method, where increasing minus lens powers are inserted monocularly to first reported slight and sustained blur.

It is common to find a reduction in accommodative ability below age-expected norms, with near vision prescriptions common even in young adults. The use of MEM[34,35] (or any preferred near retinoscopy technique) is extremely helpful when the patient is poorly or non-responsive. Frequently in ABI, the processing of questions and commands is very slow, responses delayed or unreliable, communication rambling, and possibly the patient is unable to speak. Thus, objective measurement of accommodative function by near retinoscopy is often more reliable than by subjective methods, and sometimes it is the only measurement possible where patient communication skills are unreliable or absent. I have found the following method, which has been previously described,[36,37] to be effective in determining the accommodative amplitude with many ABI patients.

Technique
Occlude one eye of the patient. Hold or fix an accommodative target (of approximately 20/30 demand) to the retinoscope as close to the line of observation as possible. Start at 40 cm from the patient, and gradually bring the retinoscope and target closer to the patient, until there is a sudden and sustained noticeable increase in magnitude of the observed lag. The distance at which this occurs is a linear measure of the objective amplitude. The same procedure is carried out with the other eye to determine if the amplitudes are essentially equal and at the level expected for the patient's age.

Accommodative stability: sustenance/fatigue
The stability of the accommodative response is often not routinely determined. However, I have found it to be an important clinical consideration with ABI patients. It is observed by monitoring the stability of the MEM or other retinoscopic lag with continued reading. Thus, determine the patient's lag of accommodation and then introduce appropriate reading material. The level of stability is an indirect measure of the patient's ability to sustain or to fatigue during a prolonged accommodative task. It is not unusual in cases of ABI to see an initial lag increase rapidly in only a brief period of time; such fatigue often manifests as symptoms of asthenopia and blur after reading for a short time.

Accommodative flexibility: inertia
Accommodative flexibility (also termed facility) is the ability to change accommodation from one target to another at different distances in space. Accommodative infacility (accommodative inflexibility or inertia) signifies a very slow or inadequate ability to change the accommodative status.[38]

Accommodative flexibility is typically assessed by having the patient observe a 20/30 optotype or group of words at a specified near distance while changing lenses monocularly or binocularly. The number of cycles of plus/minus lenses the patient can clear in one minute is recorded. Normative data has been established for both testing conditions.[39-41]

Objective measurement of accommodative facility provides the ability to observe the dynamic nature of accommodation through flippers, particularly fluctuations during testing which indicate an inability to sustain accommodation,[42] and to ensure that patients are in fact in focus when they say they are. In my experience, MEM retinoscopy can be used to assess accommodative facility by having the patient continue to read while plus and minus lenses are interposed; record the comparative speed and adequacy of the adjustment of the lag of accommodation to plus versus minus lenses, whether the adjustment is sustained, and if there is any fatigue which manifests as rapidly deteriorating response to repeated lens changes.

Other tests of factors related to accommodative function

Convergence testing should always be performed and considered in relation to accommodation function. For instance, low accommodative amplitudes and unstable accommodative accuracy for near tasks in a patient with ABI indicate that the person has significant difficulty initiating and sustaining accurate focus on a near object. Convergence is not uncommonly affected, possibly resulting in clinical measurement of convergence weakness or convergence fatigue.

Perform a normal nearpoint of convergence test, while carefully observing for binocular instability. When diplopia is reported or a deviation of one eye is observed, slowly move the target away until realignment is observed and reported. Often, in ABI of long standing, the patient will be unaware of diplopia, and there is an observable lack of binocular motor fusion. Repeat the test up to three times to determine if fatigue of convergence occurs. When the nearpoint of convergence recedes quickly, repeat the test with a pair of plus lenses, commencing at +0.75D or more if indicated on objective trials as discussed below. Very frequently, a receded or fatiguing nearpoint of convergence will be observed to improve significantly with plus lenses, indicating that the convergence deficit is secondary to an accommodative dysfunction.

In cases of apparently normal convergence, and where symptoms suggest an accommodative-convergence dysfunction, it is sometimes useful to perform the nearpoint of convergence test with a red lens before one eye, observing a penlight target binocularly. (The red lens provides a greater dissociating stimulus.) Convergence which is worse with the red lens strongly suggests a very "fragile" binocular vision system. The patient should be questioned to determine the presence of crossed or uncrossed diplopia.

Phorias (at distance and near) and fusion ranges (phoroptor, prism bar, vectograms) should also be assessed to obtain a comprehensive picture of spatial operations of accommodation and vergence.

Management of Accommodative Dysfunction

This section will first include an overview of the management of the various accommodative dysfunctions that have been previously proposed and are in current clinical use.[43,44] It will then be followed by more specific clinical management strategy.

Overview

Medications

Many ABI patients are frequently prescribed medications for conditions such as hypertension, depression, epilepsy and anxiety. These and other agents are known to affect accommodation and should be considered in cases when this function is impaired. Cooper has presented an extensive listing of the drugs that may cause or contribute to accommodative dysfunctions.[45]

Accommodative insufficiency

Accommodative insufficiency occurs when the amplitude is low or the ability to sustain accommodation is poor.[46,47] It is common in cases of whiplash[48-50] and cases of anoxia,[51,52] such as anoxic encephalopathy following severe head and/or body trauma when blood supply to the brain is temporarily compromised. It is also a common effect of myasthenia gravis.[53] Patients may have a reduced amplitude, a low positive relative accommodation measurement, and/or weak accommodative facility.

Management includes use of low plus lenses, accommodative therapy, and attention to health factors. Commonly, accommodative insufficiency is associated with accommodative fatigue, and the lag of accommodation will increase with attempted near visual tasks.

Leslie has reported five cases of accommodative insufficiency and fatigue subsequent to traumatic brain injury.[54] In most cases an initial benefit with plus lenses was reduced by a poorly dynamic accommodative system, but all patients acquired normal accommodative ability by using plus lenses combined with vision therapy.

Accommodative fatigue
(Ill-sustained accommodation)

In this condition, sustained accommodative effort results in an increasing lag and decreased facility. Management includes low plus lenses and vision therapy.

Accommodative inertia

Inertia of accommodation is a variant of accommodative infacility, as accommodation takes a relatively long time to respond to a change in stimulus. Disturbances of the cerebellar pathway may result in abnormally slow accommodative response times.[57] Inertia of accommodation is evident objectively during near retinoscopy by the patient's accommodative response to minus lenses. Typically, the response to minus lenses will take some time to commence and is quite slow in gradually reducing the lag.

Management includes plus lenses and accommodative facility therapy.

Accommodative infacility
This is a slow or inadequate response to a change in lens or target distance. Facility of accommodation may be weak despite amplitudes being relatively normal, but accommodative insufficiency and infacility commonly occur together. Typically, patients will take significantly more than one second to adjust accommodation to lenses of plus or minus power during flexibility testing.

Accommodative infacility may be encountered in the early stages of accommodative paresis or spasm, and it is important to seek a history of increased intracranial pressure or possible midbrain lesions.

Management involves accommodative facility vision therapy activities with plus lens support where indicated by testing detailed below.

Paralysis of accommodation
Paralysis, or total loss of accommodation, as distinct from insufficiency of accommodation, may result from:[56-62]

- congenital anomalies
- infection
- degenerative diseases affecting the brainstem
- diabetes
- glaucoma
- chronic alcoholism
- traumatic mydriasis
- trauma, especially motor vehicle accidents

The condition may be unilateral or bilateral. Management involves use of appropriate plus lens prescription in reading, either bifocal or progressive designs. Carefully assess pupil size (both in the light and dark) and pupil reactions. It is also advisable to probe for indications of micropsia. Clinicians should consider Adie's syndrome or a third nerve problem when significantly decreased accommodation is accompanied by a dilated pupil.

Accommodative excess
(Accommodative spasm,[63,64] pseudomyopia, ciliary spasm)
In accommodative excess, the response is greater than the stimulus de-

mand. A lead of accommodation (against movement) is seen with dynamic retinoscopy.[65] A lead of accommodation is uncommon in normal subjects; for instance an overaccommodation of 0.50D or more was seen in only 8 of 721 schoolchildren (1%) in one study.[66] Rutstein[67] described a study of 17 cases of accommodative spasm/convergence excess and found the accommodative response difficult to measure and variable with a lead of accommodation ranging between 0.75 and 5.00 diopters. Typically, the patient will have difficulty clearing monocular plus lenses in accommodative facility testing, and there will be a very low negative relative accommodation (plus to blur).

Symptoms may include asthenopia, especially frontal brow ache, and decreased vision at distance and possibly at near. Photosensitivity, poor concentration and/or diplopia may also occur. Suchoff et al. have suggested accommodative excess is caused by "an irritative lesion to the parasympathetic system."[68] The condition can be unilateral or bilateral; if unilateral, ocular trauma or inflammation should be carefully considered.

A prepresbyopic patient taking antiglaucoma drugs following trauma to the eye may also manifest accommodative spasm. Any disturbance of input to the oculomotor neurons in the midbrain may result in accommodative spasm. An accommodative spasm may be symptomatic of local inflammation as well as central nervous system lesions. The accommodative spasm may result in significant esophoria or esotropia in an individual with a high AC/A ratio. Assessment should include careful cycloplegic examination.

Management should include appropriate illumination, frequent rests from near visual tasks, and vision therapy emphasizing plus lens relaxation of accommodative effort. Scheiman and Wick have suggested a vision therapy protocol for accommodative excess.[69]

In my experience, some patients with moderate accommodative excess secondary to ABI respond to judicious application of plus lenses. This can be objectively determined by observing the lead of accommodation with MEM retinoscopy and placing plus lenses binocularly before the patient's eyes. Commence with +0.50D OU and observe if the lead reduces or changes to a lag; if so, increase plus power until no further beneficial change is observed, or there is a shift towards a lead of accommodation again. The optimal plus lens prescription is often indicated by a bright and stable reflex with low lag, or the maximum lens power which reduces the lead or optimizes the lag. Predictably, in most cases, plus lenses only increase the lead of accommodation and are contraindicated at that stage.

Cycloplegic agents may be used to reduce accommodative activity to improve distance vision, but spectacles for near and sunglasses will be necessary as well.

Convergence spasm or spasm of the near reflex

This is an infrequent clinical entity,[70] which consists of the triad of intermittent and sometimes painful episodes of sustained maximal convergence, accommodative spasm and pupil constrictions.

It may be a more extreme variation of accommodative excess. Limited abduction and severe myopia may also occur transiently. Convergence spasm is typically induced by fixation on a near object.

Clinical Strategy

It is important to correct any refractive error, even though it may be relatively small, before assessing and prescribing for accommodative dysfunction. A previously uncorrected degree of hyperopia, especially in an early presbyope, may now cause significant difficulties for a patient with ABI due to the loss of accommodative compensation. Accommodative assessment should be performed with and without this previously unimportant hyperopic correction. Similarly, a myopic prescription worn constantly prior to the brain injury may make accommodation at near more difficult post-trauma, and accommodation should be assessed with and without an habitual myopic correction.[71]

The effects on memory of CVA or TBI often result in previous spectacle prescriptions not being worn in rehabilitative care, and other rehabilitation professionals and caregivers may be unaware the patient wore spectacles prior to the brain injury. It is important to ascertain from family members or previous vision care practitioners whether or not the patient wore spectacles before the ABI, and for which functions, such as reading only, or constantly.

Similarly, the patient may not have the head or body postural control to continue to use bifocals or multifocals. This is especially so when head posture compensations have occurred subsequent to fourth or sixth nerve palsies or when the patient is in a wheelchair that has poor head support. Family members, caregivers and other rehabilitative professionals may not realize the impossibility of using a multifocal near correction in a skewed and fatigable posture in a chair or bed.

While bifocals can be considered in some cases where different prescriptions are required for distance and near tasks, it is common to find poor postural stability and possibly impaired locomotion skills in brain-injured patients. Thus, do not be too keen to prescribe bifocals for the sake of not having to change glasses. It is frequently preferable to prescribe separate distance and near corrections and possibly an intermediate prescription for music, hobbies, computer, etc. Carefully consider the visual demands of the patient through discussion with the patient, caregivers, other professionals involved in rehabilitation, and family members.[72]

It is important to provide written instructions for the patient, family members, caregivers and other professionals providing rehabilitative services as to when and for which tasks the spectacles should be worn. For instance, a mildly myopic patient with severe accommodative dysfunction may require one pair of spectacles for distance vision tasks, work unaided on the computer, and require a reading prescription for other near work. If separate prescriptions for distance and near vision are prescribed, they should be clearly identified by frame color or other marking devices. Patients with ABI frequently have short-term memory impairments which cause confusion in remembering which glasses are to be worn at different times, or even that different spectacles are available.

It is frequently necessary to use near retinoscopy to determine objectively the most appropriate lenses for near correction at the same time as assessment of accommodation. These are the lenses which result in equally low and stable lags of accommodation for both eyes. This is a useful technique for the presbyope who does not have the language and/or mental skills to respond to subjective tests to determine near reading addition, as well as the nonpresbyope who requires plus lenses due to an accommodative dysfunction secondary to acquired brain injury.

Technique
1. Using MEM retinoscopy, measure the lag of accommodation of each eye by briefly interposing plus lenses monocularly until the movement is neutralized, while the patient binocularly observes a target at the appropriate reading distance.

2. Place a pair of equal plus trial lenses over both eyes and remeasure the lag. For instance, if the patient has a lag of +1.50D OU, try +1.00D OU. In a reasonably responsive system, the "wedge" of plus may be sufficient to allow the accommodative system to respond again to the task demand, and you will see a low degree, bright and stable lag. In a poorly responsive system, +1.00D OU may still leave a large and variable lag. This indicates that more plus (e.g. +1.50D OU) should be used. Basically, you are searching for the plus lenses that produce a lag of accommodation which is equal for the two eyes, stable, bright, and of the order of +0.25D to +0.50D OU. In my experience, a low lag of this magnitude with lens help will result in stable, comfortable and efficient ac-

commodative function with extended near visual demands. A lag of +0.75D or more usually results in an increasing lag with time (i.e., accommodative fatigue) and consequently reduced near vision performance.

3. However, in many cases of ABI, the accommodative response to plus lens assistance is weak, and even the use of increasing plus may show a continuing lag of accommodation. This suggests a need for associated vision therapy in order to redevelop more responsive and flexible accommodative functioning. In such circumstances, it is acceptable, in my experience, to use a temporary large reading addition for the short term, while employing vision therapy to retrain accommodation. As the accommodative response improves, the near plus addition may be reduced.

4. If the lags are unequal through the subjective distance prescription and a near add is indicated, reassess the distance prescription and then consider unequal adds. When the lags are unequal, even with trial binocular plus which reduces the lag to a small level, use unequal trial lenses while performing MEM retinoscopy to find the combination that produces the desired effect described above. It is surprising how sensitive some patients are to small differences in the add, and how often they can verbally express, or demonstrate by facial expression, the most suitable lens combination.

Accommodative lags may be unequal for the two eyes in unilateral or even bilateral paresis. Especially in the early stages of an acquired fourth or sixth cranial nerve palsy, the disturbance to binocular function often disturbs the accommodative response of one or both eyes, thus resulting in unequal or variable lags of accommodation. Reading glasses may be necessary in the short term to enable the patient to clearly read. Of course, the diplopia of a sixth nerve palsy would also have to be considered, as must the cyclotorsional diplopia and blur in downgaze of a fourth nerve palsy. It is my belief that the accommodative dysfunction in these paretic conditions is a consequence of a dysfunctional convergence system. It is not unusual to find accommodation returning to a more normal function as the paresis resolves.

A third nerve palsy frequently affects pupil size and accommodation, and the best lens for each eye must be considered separately, as well as whether binocular function is possible; fortuitously, the acquired ptosis of a third nerve palsy may act as a natural occluder and prevent diplopia in the short term. Aberrant regeneration of the third nerve may result in pupillary abnormalities and accommodative excess.[73]

In my experience, a small pupil usually accompanies excessive accommodative effort, and a large pupil often accompanies a high or easily fatigued lag in ABI.

When a patient complains of diplopia, it is important to determine if the problem is actually two separate images, or blur and ghosting which the patient describes as double vision. Ask the patient: " Do you see two separate pictures like this (holding your hands up and apart), or do you see blurred pictures on top of each other like ghosting on television (holding your two hands over each other)?" If the patient reports two separate images, you can ask where the two images are and hold your hands separated horizontally, vertically and obliquely to identify horizontal, vertical or oblique diplopia. The images may be both blurred and diplopic, as in convergence dysfunction associated with accommodative dysfunction, or a fourth or sixth nerve palsy with associated blur.

Convergence dysfunction commonly occurs secondary to accommodative dysfunction, and any complaints of blur require careful testing of convergence function. It is important to repeat the pushup test of convergence, because the nearpoint of convergence may rapidly recede over two or three trials in cases of convergence fatigue in ABI.

Blunt trauma to the eye often results in initial miosis and accommodative spasm; the pupil may change to a traumatic mydriasis, and while accommodation often can return to normal over the following months, in a severe injury accommodative paresis may result. Any traumatic iritis or iridocyclitis will decrease accommodation.

In any frontal trauma where accommodative deficiencies are manifested, sinus involvement should be considered.

Where severe body trauma has occurred, as in a fall from height, or head-on road trauma, even though there is no direct ocular trauma, look carefully for signs of macula edema or a macular hole that may affect accommodation.

Vision Therapy for Accommodation in Acquired Brain Injury

Vision therapy to rehabilitate accommodative disorders is directed to improve accommodative amplitude, develop more normal and sustained accuracy of accommodative response for near targets, and improve speed and accuracy of accommodative dynamics. Repetition of vision therapy techniques is aimed at developing automatic and sustained accommodative function. It is also important to develop "flexibility" between accommodation and vergence functions, so that small changes in vergence do not cause large changes in accommodation.

Reprogramming accommodative function through vision therapy requires a number of conditions:[74]

- a visual environment
- repetition, feedback and reinforcement
- multisystem involvement
- active patient participation
- problem-solving task demand

Vision therapy has been shown to be an effective treatment to improve accommodative facility, speed of accommodative response, and accommodative amplitude, as well as eliminating accommodative spasm.[75-80] Vision therapy to treat accommodative dysfunctions in acquired brain injury has been described by a number of authors,[81] but to date there has not been a comprehensive description of the principles underlying therapy, effective activities, and expected duration of treatment and outcomes.

Thomas has suggested accommodation should be treated early in a program of vision therapy, in parallel with eye movements, fixation, movement and balance.[82] This would be followed by development of equal monocular skills; monocular function in a binocular field and antisuppression work; fusion development; fusion ranges and accommodative-convergence flexibility; and perceptual therapy.

Commence with accommodative skills therapy monocularly, then work biocularly (use monocular function in a binocular field, or dissociating prism to create two images with different accommodative demands) or alternately (switch lenses from right to left eye with the other eye occluded) where possible, then proceed to binocular accommodative therapy.

Summary

Accommodative dysfunctions are one of the most common sequelae of mild head injuries, yet are often undetected despite causing significant interference with the comfort and efficiency of a person's ability to carry out activities such as reading and computer work. Moderate to severe brain injuries acquired as a result of stroke, trauma, drug overdoses, and poisoning, often cause severe dysfunctions of accommodation.

Any accommodative dysfunction in ABI has the potential to limit performance of activities of daily living and the quality of life of that person. At the same time, the limitations on visual performance caused by an accommodative dysfunction can significantly retard progress in other rehabilitation, particularly cognitive, occupational and speech therapies.

Difficulties in acquiring visual information resulting from an accommodative dysfunction can also detract from visual information processing and association, when attention is inordinately directed to the lower-order act of focusing and away from higher-order processing. As a result, neuropsychological assessment of a person with an acquired brain injury and associated visual deficits may result in an invalid assessment of cognitive abilities and potential.

An optometrist can assist a person with an ABI to reach full visual potential through careful and reliable assessment of accommodation, in the process of comprehensive evaluation of all visual and ocular factors. The specific accommodative dysfunctions commonly resulting from ABI have been detailed, and valid testing protocols described to enable an optometrist to determine accommodative function in a person with compromised brain abilities, even when language and processing deficits are severe. Options for management of these accommodative problems, including lenses and vision therapy, have been detailed with specific guidelines for management of many of the unusual presentations commonly encountered in treating patients with ABI.

Optometrists can make a significant difference to the quality of life of many people with ABI, where so often the visual deficit is undetected despite previous assessments. The changes in visual performance and life skills are often dramatic and very satisfying for the patient and optometrist.

References

1. Phillips SR, Stark L. Blur: a sufficient accommodative stimulus. Doc Ophthalmol 1977;43:65-89.
2. Heath GG. The influence of visual acuity on accommodative responses of the eye. Am J Optom 1956;33:513-24.
3. Fincham E. The accommodative reflex and its stimulus. Br J Ophthalmol 1951;35:381-93.
4. Rosenfield M, Gilmartin B. Effect of target proximity on the open-loop accommodative response. Optom Vis Sci 1990;67:74-9.
5. Wick B, Currie D. Dynamic demonstration of proximal vergence and proximal accommodation. Optom Vis Sci 1991;68:163-7.
6. Rosenfield M, Ciuffreda KJ. Proximal and cognitively-induced accommodation. Ophthal Physiol Opt 1990;10:252-6.
7. Zost, MG. Diagnosis and management of visual dysfunction in cerebral injury. In: Maino DM, ed. Diagnosis and Management of Special Populations. Santa Ana, CA: Optometric Extension Program Foundation, 2001:81-84. (Originally published by Mosby, 1995.)
8. Peachey G. Minimum attention model for understanding the development of visual function. Behav Optom 1991 Jan-Feb:10-19.
9. Howell ER. The differential diagnosis of accommodation/convergence disorders. Behav Optom 1991; Jan-Feb:20-6.

10. Gianutsos R et al. Rehabilitative optometric services for survivors of acquired brain injury. Arch Phys Med Rehabil 1988;69:573-8.
11. Kowal L. Ophthalmic manifestations of head injury. Aust NZ J Ophthalmol 1992;20:35-40.
12. Al-Qurainy IA. Convergence insufficiency and failure of accommodation following midfacial trauma. Br Orthopt J 1995;32:71-5.
13. Harrison RJ. Loss of fusional vergence with partial loss of accommodative convergence and accommodation following head injury. Binoc Vis 1987;2:93-100.
14. Roca PD. Ocular manifestations of whiplash injuries. Ann Ophthalmol 1972;4:63-73.
15. Ohtsuka K, Maeskawa H, Takeda M, Uede N, Chiba S. Accommodation and convergence insufficiency with left middle cerebral artery occlusion. Am J Ophthalmol 1988;106:60-4.
16. Gilmartin B. A review of the role of sympathetic innervation of the ciliary muscle in ocular accommodation. Ophthal Physiol Opt 1986;6:23-37.
17. Rosenfield M. Accommodation. In: Zadnick K, ed. The Ocular Examination. Philadelphia PA: WB Saunders, 1997:88-9.
18. Snell RS, Lemp MA. Clinical Anatomy of the Eye. 2nd ed. Malden MA: Blackwell Science, 1998.
19. Wick B, Hall P. Relation among accommodative facility, lag, and amplitude in elementary school children. Am J Optom Physiol Opt 1987; 64:593-8.
20. Rouse MW, Hutter RF, Shiftlett R. A normative study of the accommodative lag in elementary school children. Am J Optom Physiol Opt 1984;61:693-7.
21. Ciuffreda KJ, Kenyon RV. Accommodative vergence and accommodation in normals, amblyopes and strabismics. In: Schor CM, Ciuffreda KJ, eds. Vergence Eye Movements: Basic and Clinical Aspects. Boston: Butterworths Publishers, 1983:101-74.
22. Whitefoot H, Charman WN. Dynamic retinoscopy and accommodation. Ophthal Physiol Opt 1992;12:8-17.
23. Ong J, Schuchert J. Dissociated versus monocular cross cylinder method. Am J Optom Arch Am Acad Optom 1972;49:762-4.
24. Rosenfield M, Ciuffreda KJ. Accommodative responses to conflicting stimuli. J Opt Soc Am A 1991;8:422-7.
25. Williamson-Noble FA. A possible fallacy in the use of the cross-cylinder. Br J Ophthalmol 1943;27:1-2.
26. Rouse MW, London R, Allen DC. An evaluation of the monocular estimate method of dynamic retinoscopy. Am J Optom Physiol Opt 1982;59:234.
27. McKee GW. Reliability of monocular estimate method retinoscopy. Optom Mon 1981;72:30-1.
28. Locke LC, Somers W. A comparison study of dynamic retinoscopy techniques. Optom Vis Sci 1989;66:540-44.
29. Jackson TW, Goss DA. Variation and correlation of clinical tests of accommodative function in a sample of school-age children. J Am Optom Assoc 1991;62:857-66.
30. Hofstetter HW. A comparison of Duane's and Donders' table of the amplitude of accommodation. Am J Optom Arch Am Acad Optom 1944;21:345-63.
31. Borish IM. Clinical Refraction. 3rd ed. Chicago: Professional Press, 1970.
32. Hofstetter HW. A useful table for age and amplitude. Optom World 1950;38:42-5.
33. Woehrle MB, Frantz KA. Accommodative amplitude estimation: can we substitute the pull-away for the push-up method? J Optom Vis Dev 1997;28:246-50.
34. Rutstein RP, Fuhr PD, Swiatocha J. Comparing the amplitude of accommodation determined objectively and subjectively. Optom Vis Sci 1993;70:496-500.
35. Haynes HM. Clinical observations with dynamic retinoscopy. Optom Wkly 1960;51:2243-6, 2306-9.

36. Brookman KE. A retinoscopic method of assessing accommodative performance of young human infants. J Am Optom Assoc 1981;52:865-9.

37. Hokoda SC, Ciuffreda KJ. Measurement of accommodative amplitude in amblyopia. Ophthal Physiol Opt 1982;2:205-12.

38. Duke-Elder S, Abrams D. Ophthalmic optics and refraction. In: Duke-Elder S, ed. System of Ophthalmology. St Louis: Mosby, 1970;5:451-86.

39. Garzia R, Richman J. Accommodative facility: a study of young adults. J Am Optom Assoc 1982;53:821-24.

40. Zellers J, Alpert T, Rowe M. A review of the literature and a normative study of accommodative infacility. J Am Optom Assoc 1984;55:31-7.

41. Levine S, Ciuffreda K, Selenow A et al. Clinical assessment of accommodative facility in symptomatic and asymptomatic individuals. J Am Optom Assoc 1985;56:286-90.

42. Gallaway M, Scheiman M. Assessment of accommodative facility using MEM retinoscopy. J Am Optom Assoc 1990; 61:36-9.

43. Duane A. Anomalies of accommodation clinically considered. Trans Am Ophthalmol Soc 1915;1:386-400.

44. Scheiman M, Wick B. Clinical Management of Binocular Vision. Philadelphia PA: JB Lippincott, 1994:339-78.

45. Cooper J. Accommodative dysfunction. In: Amos J, ed. Diagnosis and Management in Vision Care. Boston: Butterworth-Heinemann, 1987.

46. Harrison RJ. Loss of fusional vergence with partial loss of accommodative convergence and accommodation following head injury. Binocular Vision 1987;2:93-100.

47. Wescott V. Concerning accommodative asthenopia following head injury. Am J Ophthalmol 1936;19:385-91.

48. Burke JP, Orton HP, West J, Strachan IM, Hockey MS, Ferguson DG. Whiplash and its effect on the visual system. Graefe's Arch Clin Exper Ophthalmol 1992;230:335-9.

49. Girling WNM. Whiplash injuries: their effect on accommodative convergence, peripheral and central field, together with treatment used. XVIII Concilium Ophthalmologicum Belgium 1958;2:1550-6.

50. Roca PD. Ocular manifestations of whiplash injuries. Ann Ophthalmol 1972;4:65-73.

51. Berens C, Stark E. Studies in ocular fatigue. IV. Fatigue of accommodation, experimental and clinical observations. Am J Ophthalmol 1932;15:527-42.

52. Bietti G. Effect of increased or decreased oxygen supply in some ophthalmic diseases. Arch Ophthalmol 1953;49:449-513.

53. Manson N, Stark G. Defects of near vision in myasthenia gravis. Lancet 1965;1:935-37.

54. Leslie S. Optometric management of accommodative-convergence dysfunction in acquired brain injury. Behav Optom (in press).

55. Kawasaki T, et al. Slow accommodation release with a cerebellar lesion. Br J Ophthalmol 1993;77:678.

56. Tornqvist G. Paralysis of accommodation. Acta Ophthalmol 1971;49:702-6.

57. Duke-Elder S, Scott GI. Neuro-ophthalmology. In: Duke-Elder S, ed. System of Ophthalmology. St Louis: Mosby, 1971;12:698-703.

58. Hofstetter HW. Factors involved in low amplitude cases. Am J Optom 1942;19:279-89.

59. Mortada A. Self-curable iridodonesis after blunt ocular injury. Bull Ophthalmol Soc Egypt 1970;63:323-4.

60. Blatt N. Weakness of accommodation. Arch Ophthalmol 1931;5:362-63.

61. Duane A. Anomalies of the accommodation clinically considered. Trans Am Ophthalmol Soc 1915;1:386-402.

62. Dralands L, Adrianesseus L. Persistent isolated paralysis of accommodation in young people. Bull Soc Belgian Ophthalmol 1978;182:42-50.

63. Bohlmann BJ, France TD. Persistent accommodative spasm nine years after head trauma. J Clin Neuro-Ophthalmol 1987;7:129-31.

64. Smith JL. Accommodative spasm versus spasm of the near reflex. J Clin Neuro-Ophthalmol 1987;7:132-34.

65. Griffin JR. Binocular Anomalies: Procedures for Vision Therapy. 2nd ed. Chicago: Professional Press, 1982: 381-82.

66. Rouse MW, Hutter RF, Shiflett R. A normative study of the accommodative lag in elementary schoolchildren. Am J Optom Physiol Opt 1984;61:693-97.

67. Rutstein RP, Daum KM, Amos JF. Accommodative spasm: a study of 17 cases. J Am Optom Assoc 1988;59:527-38.

68. Suchoff IB, Gianutsos G, Ciuffreda KJ, Groffman S. Vision impairment related to acquired brain injury. In: B Silverstone, ed. The Lighthouse Handbook on Vision Impairment and Vision Rehabilitation. New York, NY: Oxford University Press, 2000:527.

69. Scheiman M, Wick B. Clinical Management of Binocular Vision. Philadelphia PA: JB Lippincott, 1994:360-66.

70. Miller NR. Nuclear and infranuclear ocular motility disorders. In: Walsh FB, Hoyt WF, Miller NR. Clinical Neuro-Ophthalmology. 4th ed. Baltimore: Williams and Wilkins, 1991:528-35.

71. Suchoff IB, Gianutsos R, Ciuffreda KJ, Groffman S. Vision impairment related to acquired brain injury. In: Silverstone B, Lang MA, Rosenthal BP, Faye EE, eds. The Lighthouse Handbook On Vision Impairment And Vision Rehabilitation, Vol I. New York: Oxford University Press, 2000:549-73.

72. Suchoff IB, Gianutsos R. Rehabilitative optometric interventions for the acquired brain injured patient. In: Grabois M, Garrison SJ, Hart KA, and Lehmkuhl DL, eds. Physical Medicine and Rehabilitation: The Complete Approach. Boston: Blackwell, 1999.

73. Miller NR, Newman NJ. The Essentials–Walsh and Hoyt's Clinical Neuro-Ophthalmology, 5th ed. Baltimore: Williams and Wilkins, 1999.

74. Cohen AH. Optometric rehabilitative therapy. In: LJ Press, ed. Applied Concepts in Vision Therapy. St Louis: Mosby,1997:278-86.

75. The 1986/1987 AOA Future of Visual Development/Performance Task Force. The efficacy of optometric vision therapy. J Am Optom Assoc 1988;59:95-105.

76. Daum K. Accommodative insufficiency. Am J Optom Physiol Opt 1983;60:352-59.

77. Hoffman L, Cohen A, Feuer G. Effectiveness of non-strabismic optometric vision training in a private practice. Am J Optom Arch Am Acad Optom 1973;50:813-16.

78. Liu JS, Lee M, Jang J et al. Objective assessment of accommodative orthoptics: 1. Dynamic insufficiency. Am J Optom Physiol Opt 1979;56:285-91.

79. Bobier WR, Sivak JG. Orthoptic treatment of subjects showing slow accommodative responses. Am J Optom Physiol Opt 1983;60:678-87.

80. Rouse MW. Management of binocular anomalies: efficacy of vision therapy in the treatment of accommodative deficiencies. Am J Optom Physiol Opt 1987;64:415-20.

81. Suter PS. Rehabilitation and management of visual dysfunction following traumatic brain injury. In: Ashley MJ, Krych DK, eds. Traumatic Brain Injury Rehabilitation. Boca Raton, FL: CRC Press, 1995:198-220.

82. Thomas JA. Head trauma: traumatic brain injury-visual dysfunction and optometric rehabilitation. Presented at International Congress of Behavioural Optometry, Sydney, Australia, April, 1994.

Oculomotor Consequences of Acquired Brain Injury

Kenneth J. Ciuffreda, O.D., Ph.D.
Ying Han, M.D., Ph.D.
Neera Kapoor, O.D., M.S.
Irwin B. Suchoff, O.D., D.O.S.

Introduction

Acquired brain injury (ABI) affects relatively large regions of the brain due to the pervasive nature of the primary insult. Hence, the consequences are broad and can adversely affect the sensory, motor, perceptual, cognitive, psychological and/or behavioral states.[1-7]

One such area of interest, and in which many patients with ABI are affected, is the oculomotor system.[1,2,6-9] The oculomotor neural network is extensive, thus leading to multiple oculomotor and related subsystem deficits from a single cranial insult (Table 1).[2] Furthermore, many of the same areas of the brain contribute to multiple oculomotor functions. For example, the frontal, parietal, and cerebellar regions each participate in both saccadic and pursuit neural control.[10] The resultant oculomotor dysfunctions, either in isolation or more typically in conjunction with deficits in the other non-oculomotor systems mentioned earlier, can clearly have adverse educational, social, and economic impact on the affected individual, as well as on the family members who extend their care.

In this chapter, we will review the etiology of ABI and its oculomotor consequences. In addition, therapeutic paradigms and their outcomes will be discussed.

Traumatic Brain Injury (TBI)

According to Title VII of the U.S. Public Health Service Act of 1994, "the term 'traumatic brain injury' means acquired injury to the brain. Such term does not include brain dysfunction by congenital or degenerative disorders, nor birth trauma, but may include brain injuries caused by anoxia due to near drowning." Furthermore, according to the National Center for Health Statistics,[11] there are 8 million head injuries per year with 1.5 million considered to be "major." These injuries result in 100,000 deaths per year, and as many as 700,000 victims require hospitalization. About 60% of the TBI patients do not return to the workforce, thus resulting in a national economic loss of 4 billion dollars.[4]

Table 1. Common Functional and Symptomatic Consequences of ABI on the Oculomotor and Accommodative Systems	
Component	Consequence
Vergence	Diplopia Reading problems Asthenopia Headaches Blurred print Closing or covering one eye
Accommodation	Focusing problems Headaches Inability to maintain clear vision when reading and studying Squinting both eyes
Strabismus	Closing or covering one eye Diplopia Head tilting or turning Impaired spatial judgment
Version	Difficulty in tracking objects Skipping, rereading, and reversing words Loss of place when reading

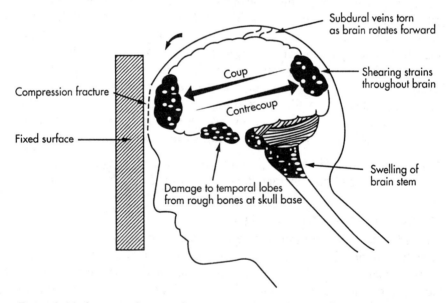

Figure 1. Mechanisms of coup and contrecoup injuries (Reprinted with permission from Zost[4]).

The etiology of TBI can perhaps best be visualized and explained by Figure 1.[4] With a single direct blow to the skull, brain injury may occur in two opposing regions. At the point of impact, the underlying brain tissue receives contusion. This is referred to as coup injury. However, due to the differential biomechanical dynamics between the brain and skull, the brain region opposite to the direct impact (as well as other areas) may also sustain damage due to stretching/shearing of the brain, ruptured blood vessels, and/or physical contact with the rough and irregular inner surface of the skull as the brain is rapidly and transiently shifted within the fixed cranium. This is referred to as contrecoup injury. In addition, the individual may develop cerebral edema, causing global compressive effects on the brain itself. Hence, multiple noncontiguous areas of the brain can be damaged following a single and discrete blow to the skull.

Oculomotor Consequences

As mentioned earlier, the oculomotor consequences of TBI are extensive and may affect many diverse subsystems, each with specific functions, and hence compromise important daily tasks such as reading. This is evident from inspection of Table 2.[2] Present are dynamic abnormalities such as nystagmus and static abnormalities such as strabismus. In addition to the oscillopsia, diplopia, and oculomotor tracking problems which are present and directly related to the eye movement system per se, there may also be other problems such as blur and spatial difficulties, in addition to the more generalized phenomena of headaches and asthenopia (Table 1).[2] When these oculomotor-related problems are combined with the other possible sensory, motor, cognitive, etc. deficits that may be present, the resultant challenge in the home and workplace can be enormous for the patient.

Table 2.
Some Oculomotor Changes Associated with Traumatic Brain Injury

- Downbeat nystagmus
- Impaired overall oculomotor control
- Acute vertigo with head movement
- Reduced fusional vergence ranges (with or without normal nearpoint of convergence)
- Divergence paralysis
- Spasm of the near reflex
- Multiple oculomotor nerve palsies/noncomitant strabismus (fracture of head or orbital bones)
- Mechanical restriction of upward gaze (blow-out fracture)
- Fourth nerve palsy (blunt frontal-area injury)
- Strabismus
- Internuclear ophthalmoplegia

Oculomotor Rehabilitation

There have only been a few reports in the literature related to oculomotor rehabilitation in TBI patients. This has run the gamut from simple, repetitive eye tracking in the laboratory[12-15] and home[16] environments to more

Table 3. Clinical Oculomotor Improvements Following Vision Therapy for Head Trauma	Table 4. Laboratory Oculomotor Therapy Effects in Brain-Injured Patients (n = 22)

• Reduced exophoria at near
• Closer nearpoint of convergence
• Increased positive fusional range
• Improved King-Devick saccade test
• Concurrent elimination of diplopia and/or blur
	• Faster rate of improvement
	   saccades 4.5x
	   optokinetic nystagmus 3.0x
	   pursuit 2.5x
	• Higher level of improvement
	• Some oculomotor subsystem transfer

conventional and integrated sensory, motor, perceptual and attentional clinical optometric paradigms[6-8,17,18] to simple fusional training.[19]

All rehabilitation resulted in oculomotor improvements. The clinical findings in one study[17] are presented in Table 3. Clearly, improvements in both versional and vergence aspects, with concomitant elimination of symptoms, were found. The laboratory findings in another study[14] are presented in Table 4. There was multiple system improvement and transfer with simple oculomotor training, as well as a more rapid and higher level of improvement than found in the control patients followed during their natural recovery period (Figure 2).[14] And, in an extensive case report,[8] a progressive level of oculomotor improvement was found with conventional vision therapy; further improvement was documented with the prescription of base-in prisms to reduce the convergence demand (Figure 3). Saccadic intrusions during fixation reduced in frequency and amplitude, and both saccadic and pursuit tracking became more accurate.

Stroke

Approximately 500,000 individuals in the United States sustain a stroke each year.[20] It is the leading cause of chronic disability, and the third leading cause of death in the U.S. adult elderly population[21]. However, about 50% of stroke victims return to the workplace either unimpaired or with only mild disability.[22]

The etiology of stroke is twofold,[22] with both related to reduction of the high oxygen requirement of brain tissue.[23] First, it can be of an ischemic nature. This could result from hypertensive narrowing of the arteries, an embolism or artherosclerotic plaque formation. Second, it can be of a hemorrhagic nature. This could result from a ruptured blood vessel, an aneurysm or arteriovenous malformation. Due to similarities in the pathogenesis of TBI and stroke, there is considerable overlap in the ocular and visual symptoms. However, due to the hemispheric specialization of the brain (with the left side dominating speech and language, and the right

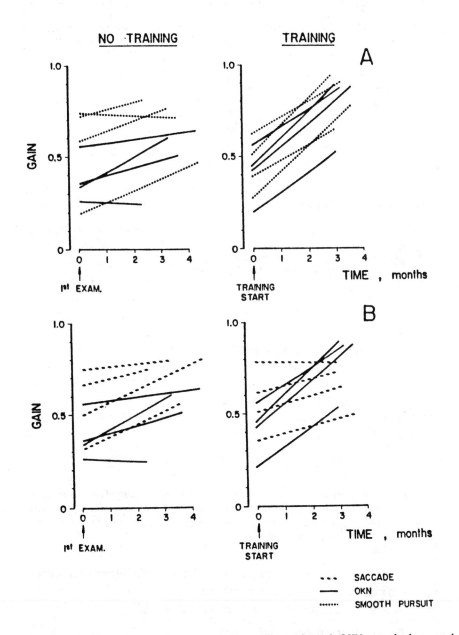

Figure 2. The gain change of contralateral saccades, ipsilateral OKN smooth phase, and smooth pursuit when subjects were trained in optokinetic movements. Each straight line represents one patient through the follow-up period. Comparison of gain trend in the various patients between (A) saccades and OKN smooth phase, and (B) saccades and smooth pursuit. (Reprinted with permission from Ron[14])

A. Pre - VT

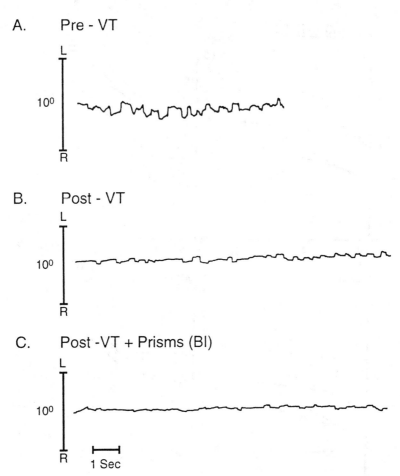

B. Post - VT

C. Post -VT + Prisms (BI)

1 Sec

Figure 3. The improvement in fixation in a patient who had a nonstrabismic anomaly of binocular vision: (A) the objective recording of fixation of the right eye before vision therapy, (B) after vision therapy, and (C) after vision therapy with the addition of compensatory prisms. (Reprinted with permission from Ciuffreda et al[8]).

side dominating visual processing and spatial aspects), significant differences will also be evident with respect to the primary dysfunction, depending upon which hemisphere is more severely damaged.

Oculomotor Consequences

As with TBI, the possible oculomotor consequences of stroke are both numerous and diverse (Table 5).[24-34] A variety of subtle oculomotor findings is evident. In the clinic examination, approximately 15% of the patients manifest versional dysfunction and 40% exhibit reduced vergence ability.[35] This includes deficits in fixational, saccadic, pursuit and vestibular

Table 5.
Objectively-Determined Oculomotor Abnormalities in Stroke

• Saccadic overshooting contralateral (hypermetria, increased gain) and undershooting ipsilateral (hypometria, decreased gain) to side of cortical lesion

• Difficulty shifting attention (increased saccadic latency and long visual-search durations) in acute state

• Difficulty in "antisaccade" task (increased latency, reduced peak velocity, and increased errors) with frontal lesions

• Reduced saccadic scanning and exploration in hemianopic field when spatial neglect present

• Inability to sustain fixation and maintain attention when microangiopathy present

• Marginal reduction in vestibulo-ocular reflex response amplitude (reduced gain) correlated with postural instability

• Impaired reading oculomotor patterns especially into hemianopic field

• Impaired convergence

• Saccadic intrusions

function, as well as gaze limitations and vergence problems.[35-39] Once again, the oculomotor effects are global. In addition, there may be attentional shift (i.e., disengagement) difficulties, as well as nonoptimal visual scanning patterns in the presence of hemianopia. If visual neglect is present, scanning into the functionally-blind field for which the patient is unaware may be reduced; in contrast, it may be increased in the patient without visual neglect due to full awareness of the visual field loss and its resultant disabling nature.

Oculomotor Rehabilitation
Two types of oculomotor rehabilitation have been used for patients with stroke. The first consisted of conventional optometric vision therapy for fusional vergence dysfunction under static and dynamic conditions.[40,41] The second involved development of more time-optimal saccadic visual scanning and visual exploration strategies into the patient's blind hemifield.[24,42-45] Both resulted in considerable improvement.

Whiplash Injury
There are as many as 3 million whiplash injuries per year in the United States.[46] About 80% return to the workplace in the first month, and nearly 95% do so in the first year.[47] The incidence of whiplash injury ranges from 0.1 to 2.0 per thousand in the population, with 25% of these acute patients progressing to chronic symptoms.[47] Thus, the cumulative effect is 1% resulting in chronic symptoms in the general population.

The five possible etiologies of whiplash injury can be best understood in relation to the diffuse and complex nature of the primary insult, which in-

Table 6.
Objectively-Determined Oculomotor Abnormalities in Whiplash
Saccadic system • increased latency • decreased peak velocity • hypometria • difficulty in "anti-saccade" task (increased errors) and "memory guided" saccade task (increased unwanted saccades)
Pursuit system • decreased velocity gain • asymmetric pursuit and decreased velocity gain with trunk torsion
Vestibulo-optokinetic system • decreased gain of the vestibulo-ocular reflex • increased gain of the optokinetic reflex • positional nystagmus
Overall vergence system • Increased time constant for convergence and divergence
Accommodative vergence system • Increased time constant for convergence • Reduced response amplitude for convergence and divergence
Reading eye movement system • Increased number of fixations • Reduced reading rate

volves injury to the neck (i.e., musculoligamentous strain or sprain of the cervical region) by an inertial acceleration or deceleration force, but without direct head trauma or loss of consciousness.[48,49] These etiologies include:[47-53] 1) damage to small blood vessels which supply those central nervous system areas involved in oculomotor control, 2) damage to nerve roots or peripheral nerves related to axonal shearing and stretching forces in the vicinity of the III, IV, or VI cranial nerves, 3) cervical sympathetic irritation, 4) vertebrobasilar artery insufficiency and 5) disturbance of neck proprioceptive information related to the sense of head position, neck reflexes and related postural processes, and the vestibular system. As evident from above, the extensive neck proprioceptive system has direct connections with the brainstem, vestibular nuclei, cerebellum, superior colliculus and frontal eye fields, and indirect connections with the midbrain, visual cortex and parietal area; hence, it can have influence on a variety of visual, motor and spatial functions.

Oculomotor Consequences

As is true for both TBI and stroke, as a result of the complexity of neural interconnections and interactions, the oculomotor consequences of whiplash injury are both numerous and diverse[49,50,54-56] (Table 6). They include a variety of dynamic abnormalities of the saccadic, pursuit, vestibular and vergence systems; therefore, they too can have adverse impact on numerous and complex oculomotor-based vision functions, including reading.[10] The subtlety of oculomotor dysfunctions and vague symptoms, in combination with more diffuse and subtle neuroanatomical correlates, makes whiplash injury problematic and enigmatic to the medical community. However, the objective determination of these oculomotor deficits clearly demonstrates their physiological basis, especially in those patients either presenting in the acute phase or with long-term persistent complaints. Clinically, the main oculomotor dysfunctions have been related to convergence.

Oculomotor Rehabilitation

Roca[57] has reported successful oculomotor treatment in whiplash patients. This has included convergence training to improve the receded nearpoint of convergence frequently found in these patients, at times in conjunction with base-in prisms[58,59] to reduce the vergence demand, and a near add to compensate for reduced accommodative amplitude.

Future Directions

The clinical condition of acquired brain injury presents a new frontier for the optometrist as part of an interdisciplinary health care rehabilitation team. With respect to the area of eye movements, the therapeutic paradigms which have been used successfully in these patients represents, for the most part, conventional optometric vision therapy.[1,60] Future developments may include increased use of computer programs to control stimuli and quantitatively monitor and assess improvement, as well as auditory feedback to provide multisensory error information to enhance performance further.

References

1. Suchoff I, Gianutsos R. Rehabilitative optometric intervention for the adult with acquired brain injury. In: Grabois M, Garrison SJ, Hart KA, Lehmkuhl L., eds. Physical Medicine and Rehabilitation. Boston: Blackwell Science, 1999:608-21.

2. Suchoff I, Gianutsos R, Ciuffreda KJ, Groffman, S. Vision impairment related to acquired brain injury. In: Silverstone B, Lang MA, Rosenthal B, Faye EE, eds. The Lighthouse Handbook on Vision Impairment and Rehabilitation. New York: Oxford University Press, 2000:549-73.

3. Suter PS. Rehabilitation and management of visual dysfunction following traumatic brain injury. In: Ashley MJ, Krych DK, eds. Traumatic Brain Injury Rehabilitation. Boca Raton, FL: CRC Press, 1995:198-220.

4. Zost MG. Diagnosis and management of visual dysfunction in cerebral injury. In: Maino DM, ed. Diagnosis and Management of Special Populations. St. Louis: Mosby, 1995:75-134.

5. Cohen AH. Acquired visual information-processing disorders: closed-head trauma. In: Press LJ, ed. Applied Concepts in Vision Therapy. St. Louis: Mosby, 1996:165-78.

6. Morton RL. Visual dysfunction following traumatic brain injury. In: Ashley MJ, Krych DK, eds. Traumatic Brain Injury Rehabilitation. Boca Raton, FL: CRC Press, 1995:171-86.

7. Hellerstein L, Fishman B. Visual rehabilitation for patients with brain injury. In: Scheiman M, ed. Understanding and Managing Vision Deficits. Thorofare, NJ: SLACK Inc., 1997:249-81.

8. Ciuffreda KJ, Suchoff IB, Marrone MA, Ahmann, E. Oculomotor rehabilitation in traumatic brain injury. J Behav Optom 1996;7:31-8.

9. Baker RS, Epstein AD. Ocular motor abnormalities from head trauma. Surv Ophthalmol 1991;35:245-67.

10. Ciuffreda KJ, Tannen B. Eye Movement Basics for the Clinician. St. Louis: Mosby Yearbook, 1995.

11. D'Angelo CM. An overview of enhancement techniques for peripheral field loss. J Am Optom Assn 1994;64:60-70.

12. Ron S, Najenson T, Hary D, Pryworkin W. Eye movements in brain damaged patients. Scand J Rehab Med 1978;10:39-44.

13. Ron S. Plastic changes in eye movements in patients with traumatic brain injury. In: Fuchs AF, Becker W, eds. Progress in Oculomotor Research. New York: Elsevier North Holland, 1981:237-51.

14. Ron, S. Can training be transferred from one oculomotor system to another? In: Roucoux A, Crommelinck M, eds. Physiological and Pathological Aspects of Eye Movements. London: Dr. W. Junk Pub., 1982:83-8.

15. Gur S, Ron S. Training in oculomotor tracking: occupational health aspects. Israel J Med Sci 1992;28:622-28.

16. Mueller C, Koch S, Toifl K. Transient bilateral internuclear ophthalmoplegia after minor head trauma. Dev Med Child Neurol 1993;35:163-166.

17. Berne SA. Visual therapy for the traumatic brain-injured. J Optom Vis Dev 1990; 21:13-6.

18. Schlageter B, Gray B, Hall K, Shaw R, Sammet R. Incidence and treatment of visual dysfunction in traumatic brain injury. Brain Injury 1993;7:439-48.

19. Kerkhoff G, Stogerer E. Recovery of fusional convergence after systematic practice. Brain Injury 1994;8:22-6.

20. Alexander L. Pre-stroke signs and symptoms. Rev Optom 1978;8:45-53.

21. Kent T, Hart M, Shries T. Introduction to Human Disease. New York: Appleton-Crofts, 1979.

22. Kelley RE. Cerebrovascular disease. In: Weiner W.J, Goetz CG, eds. Neurology for the Non-Neurologist. Philadelphia: Lippincott, 1989:52-66.

23. Bradshaw JL, Mattingly JB. Clinical Neuropsychology Behavior and Brain Science. San Diego, CA: Academic Press,1995.

24. Pommerenke K, Markowitsch HJ. Rehabilitation training of homonymous visual field defects in patients with postgeniculate damage of the visual system. Restorative Neurol Neurosci 1989;1:47-63.

25. Schnyder H, Bassetti, C. Bilateral convergence nystagmus in unilateral dorsal midbrain stroke due to occlusion of the superior cerebellar artery. Neuro-ophthalmol 1996;16:59-63.

26. Waespe W, Mueller-Meisser E. Directional reversal of saccadic dysmetria and gain adaptivity in a patient with a superior cerebellar artery infarction. Neuro-ophthalmol 1996;16:65-74.

27. Ishiai S, Furukawa T, Tsukagoshi H. Eye fixation patterns in homonymous hemianopia and unilateral spatial neglect. Neuropsychologia 1987;25:675-79.

28. Hund M, Huber W. Eye movement behavior of patients with cerebral microangiopathy and macroangiopathy in simple visual detection tasks. Brain 1991;114:1315-21.

29. Tannen B, Ciuffreda KJ, Werner DL. A case of Wallenberg's syndrome: ocular motor abnormalities. J Am Optom Assn 1989;60:748-52.

30. Clavero M, Ciuffreda KJ, Werner DL, Tannen B. A 13-year follow-up of a case of Wallenberg's syndrome: first-person account and ocular motor abnormalities. Optometry, in press.

31. Meienberg O, Zangemeister WH, Rosenberg M, Hoyt WF, Stark L. Saccadic eye movement strategies in patients with homonymous hemianopia. Annals Neurol 1981;9:537-44.

32. Zihl J. Eye movement patterns in hemianopic dyslexia. Brain 1995;118:891-912.

33. Ciuffreda KJ, Bahill AT, Kenyon RV, Stark L. Eye movements during reading: case reports. Am J Optom Physiol Optics 1976;53:389-95.

34. Catz A, Ron S, Ring H, Solzi P, Korczyn, A. Saccadic responses in patients with hemispheric stroke. Doc. Ophthalmologica 1994;85:267-74.

35. Freeman CF, Rudge NB. The orthoptist's role in the management of stroke patients. In: Orthoptic Horizons: Transactions of the Sixth Orthoptic Congress 1987 (Sydney):333-7.

36. Freeman CF, Rudge NB. Cerebrovascular accident and the orthoptist. Br Orthopt J 1998; 45:8-18.

37. Clisby C. Visual assessment of patients with cerebrovascular accident on the elderly care wards. Br Orthopt J 1995;52:38-40.

38. Pederson RA, Troost TB. Abnormalities of gaze in cerebrovascular disease. Stroke 1981; 12:251-4.

39. Bogousslavsky J, Meienberg O. Eye movement disorders in brain stem and cerebellar stroke. Arch Neurol 1987; 44:141-48.

40. Cohen A. Visual rehabilitation of a stroke patient. J Am Optom Assn 1978; 49:830-2.

41. Cohen A, Soden R. An optometric approach to the rehabilitation of the stroke patient. J Am Optom Assn 1981;52:795-800.

42. Kerkhoff G, Munbinger U, Haaf E, Eberle-Strauss G, Stogerer E. Rehabilitation of homonymous scotomata in patients with postgeniculate damage of the visual system: saccadic compensation training. Restorative Neurol Neurosci 1992;4:245-54.

43. Webster JS, Jones S, Blanton P, Gross R, Beissel GF, Wofford JD. Visual scanning training with stroke patients. Behav Ther 1984;15:129-43.

44. Weinberg J, Diller L, Gordon WA et al. Visual scanning training effect on reading related tasks in acquired right brain injury. Arch Phys Med Rehabil 1977;58:479-86.

45. Zihl J, Werth R. Contribution to the study of "blind-sight." II. The role of specific practice for saccadic localization in patients with postgeniculate visual field defects. Neuropsychologia 1984;22:13-22.

46. Swerdlow B. Whiplash and Related Headaches. Boca Raton, FL: CRC Press, 1999.

47. Barnsley L, Lord S, Bogduk N. Whiplash injury. Pain 1994;58:283-307.

48. Fisher AJEM, Verhagen WIM, Huygen PLM. Whiplash injury: a clinical review with emphasis on neuro-otological aspects. Clin Otolaryngol 1997;22:192-201.

49. Griffiths H, Whittle J, Whelehan I, Worfolk R, Burke J. Ocular motor abnormalities following whiplash injuries. In: Orthoptics in Focus: Vision for the New Millennium. Trans. IX International Orthoptic Congress, Stockholm, 1999:153-6.

50. Hildingsson C, Wenngren BI, Bring G, Toolman G. Oculomotor problems after cervical spine injury. Acta Orthopt. Scand 1989;60:513-6.

51. Gimse R, Tjell C, Bjorgen IA, Saunte C. Disturbed eye movements after whiplash due to injuries to the posture control system. J Clin Exper Neuropsychol 1996;18:178-86.

52. Toglia JU. Acute flexion-extension injury of the neck. Neurology 1976;26:808-14.

53. Burke JP, Orton HP, West J, Strachan IM, Hockey MS, Ferguson D. Whiplash and its effect on the visual system. Graefe's Arch Clin Exper Ophthalmol 1992;230:335-9.

54. Hinoki M. Vertigo due to whiplash injury: a neurotological approach. Acta Otolaryngol (Stockholm) [suppl.] 1985;419:9-29.

55. Tjell C, Rosenhull U. Smooth pursuit neck torsion test: a specific test for cervical dizziness. Am J Otology 1998;19:76-81.

56. Mosimann UP, Muri RM, Felblinger J, Radanov BP. Saccadic eye movement disturbances in whiplash patients with persistent complaints. Brain 2000;123:828-35.

57. Roca PD. Ocular manifestations of whiplash injury. Annals Ophthalmol 1972;4:63-73.

58. Franco RF, Fells P. Ocular motility problems following road traffic accidents. Brit J Orthopt 1989;46:40-8.

59. Orton HP, Burke JP. Accommodative and convergence insufficiency following whiplash injuries. Brit Orthopt J 1993;50:19-21.

60. Kapoor N, Ciuffreda KJ. Vision disturbances following traumatic brain injury. Current Treatment Options in Neurol, in press.

Vision Therapy to Treat Binocular Vision Disorders After Acquired Brain Injury: Factors Affecting Prognosis

Mitchell Scheiman, O.D.
Michael Gallaway, O.D.

Introduction

During the past decade, optometrists have become more involved in the management of vision problems associated with acquired brain injury (ABI).[1-5] Binocular vision disorders have been reported to be among the most common vision problems occurring in this population.[2,6-8] For example, Gianutsos et al.[2] performed a vision evaluation on a population of 55 severely brain-injured individuals in a long-term rehabilitation facility. Thirty-six of the 55 subjects failed some aspect of the vision screening and were referred for a complete optometric evaluation. Twenty-six of the 36 subjects referred were evaluated by the optometrist. The two most common problems found were binocular vision disorders (19/26) and accommodative disorders (18/26). Cohen et al.[6] found convergence insufficiency in 38% of acute ABI patients and in 42% in patients re-evaluated three years after traumatic brain injury. More recently, Suchoff et al.[8] examined 62 brain-injured patients who resided in extended care facilities and found a high occurrence of exodeviations (41.9%) including convergence insufficiency, intermittent and constant exotropia, and vertical deviations (9.7%). There have also been reports on the treatment of binocular vision problems using lenses, prisms, occlusion and vision therapy.[1, 9-20] These reports, all of which were case studies, suggest that treatment can be effective in relieving patient symptoms and improving binocular function. However, it is also apparent from these case studies that the treatment of binocular vision problems after ABI is one of the more challenging aspects of optometric practice.

After reviewing these case studies, it is clear that the current literature lacks an organized presentation of the various factors that should be considered when determining the potential effectiveness of vision therapy for the treatment of binocular vision disorders after ABI. Only Krohel, Anderson and Candler discuss patient characteristics that affected prognosis in their case studies. Krohel[15] reported that response to convergence exercises was variable, often incomplete, and unpredictable. He found that patients without serious neurologic sequelae responded slightly better than those with serious neurologic involvement. However, success could not be reliably predicted on an individual basis from the type or severity of trauma. Also, the severity of the convergence problem did not positively correlate with the severity of the head trauma. Anderson[10] listed binocular status before the head injury, the patient's age, and the time elapsed after injury as important issues to consider. Candler[9] suggested that the intelligence of the patient before ABI is of utmost importance for prognosis.

Several authors have discussed determination of prognosis for treatment of binocular vision problems not associated with ABI. Flom[21] identified three characteristics that affect the treatment prognosis: 1) the direction of the deviation, 2) its frequency, and 3) the status of correspondence (anomalous or normal correspondence). Ludlam[22] reported on the results of vision therapy/orthoptics for 149 comitant strabismics. He found that a positive outcome was related to motivation on the part of the patient or guardian, consistent attendance, size of the deviation, age of onset of the strabismus, frequency of the deviation, and direction of the deviation. Caloroso and Rouse[23] stressed the importance of considering the patient's health profile, prior treatment, and patient or parent/guardian attitudes. They suggested that the presence of associated or progressive neurological disease may reduce the potential for establishing normal binocular vision. Caloroso and Rouse also emphasized that the patient (and parent or guardian) participating in a binocular vision program should have sufficient physical and mental stamina to comply with the demands of the therapy. This last point is particularly relevant to patients with ABI. In summary, these authors suggested that the following factors lead to a more positive prognosis: 1) intermittent deviation, 2) exodeviation, 3) comitant deviation, 4) normal correspondence, 5) presence of stereopsis, 6) late onset strabismus, 7) strong motivation to pursue treatment, 8) absence of progressive neurological disease, and 9) physical and mental stamina to participate in treatment.

Prognostic Factors

Based on a review of the literature and our experience with our own patients, we developed a list of potentially important prognostic factors. Table 1 lists the prognostic factors that we believe should be taken into consideration if vision therapy is being considered as a treatment approach for an ABI patient.

The objective of this chapter is to review the factors that can influence prognosis for the use of vision therapy to treat binocular vision problems

```
┌────────────────────────────────────────────────────────────┐
│                         Table 1.                            │
│            Potentially Important Prognostic Findings         │
│                                                              │
│   Cognitive Issues                                           │
│              Developmental level                             │
│              Motivation                                      │
│              Physical and mental stamina                     │
│              Memory                                          │
│              Cognitive status                                │
│              Visual information processing                   │
│              Verbal/communication skills                     │
│                                                              │
│   Characteristics of the Binocular Disorder                  │
│              Magnitude of deviation                          │
│              Direction of deviation                          │
│              Presence of a vertical deviation                │
│              Presence of a cyclodeviation                    │
│              Comitancy                                       │
│              Stereopsis                                      │
│              Presence of a sensory fusion disruption syndrome│
│                                                              │
│   Accommodative Function                                     │
│              Low amplitude of accommodation                  │
│              Unequal accommodative amplitudes                │
│                                                              │
│   Oculomotor Function                                        │
│              Saccadic dysfunction                            │
│              Pursuit dysfunction                             │
│                                                              │
│   Visual Field Loss                                          │
└────────────────────────────────────────────────────────────┘
```

after ABI. We present a series of nine case studies to demonstrate the effect of some of these factors on treatment outcome.

Method

We reviewed patient care files from 1996–1999 at the Pennsylvania College of Optometry, Binocular Vision Service and from our private practices. Records were selected if the patient had a binocular vision problem, was symptomatic, had a history of ABI, and completed a vision therapy program to treat the binocular vision disorder. We carefully reviewed the records of both successful and unsuccessful vision therapy cases to identify factors that appeared to contribute to the final outcome. Nine cases were chosen. We believe they are representative of ABI patients optometrists generally encounter in a private practice setting rather than the type of patient seen in a rehabilitation hospital who may have more severe problems.

Each case is described and reviewed to analyze retrospectively various parameters that may have either positively or negatively affected the outcome. Pre- and post-vision therapy examination findings are listed for all patients after each case report.

CASE REPORTS

Case One

History

TM, a 32-year-old white male, was struck on the back of the head with a piece of concrete weighing 150 lbs. Although he did not lose consciousness, he was evaluated at the emergency room. He was released after treatment of the wound. Since that time, he has noted blurred vision and frequent headaches after short periods of reading. He also reported intermittent horizontal diplopia after reading more than 15 minutes.

Significant clinical findings

We examined TM nine months after the head injury. At that time he was wearing soft contact lenses with a prescription of OD -2.50D and OS -2.50D. Visual acuity (with correction) at distance and near was 6/6 (20/20) OD, OS and OU. The cover test revealed orthophoria at 20 feet and a $10-12^\Delta$ intermittent alternating exotropia at near (deviated 10 percent of the time). He had 20 seconds of arc stereopsis and random-dot stereopsis. The nearpoint of convergence was receded with a break at 15 cm and a recovery at 22 cm. Step vergence ranges at near were base-in $X/14/12^\Delta$ and base-out $X/18/12^\Delta$. TM was able to complete 8 cycles per minute (cpm) with vergence facility testing (12^Δ BO/3^Δ BI) having some difficulty regaining fusion with 12^Δ base-out. The amplitude of accommodation was 5D in each eye and he was able to complete 8 cpm with binocular accommodative facility.

Diagnosis

Convergence insufficiency, accommodative insufficiency

Treatment

A vision therapy program was recommended and followed the sequence of Scheiman and Wick [24] for convergence insufficiency and accommodative insufficiency.

Outcome

TM required 11 office visits to complete the vision therapy program. At the reevaluation he could now read for as long as necessary without headaches or eyestrain.

Factors affecting outcome

In this case the outcome was excellent, and the result was achieved in a very short period of time. In fact, the number of required vision therapy sessions was typical of that required for adults with convergence insufficiency in the general population without ABI.[24] The brain injury did not impact on his cognitive skills, and he was highly motivated to regain comfortable vision. The characteristics of the binocular and accommodative problems were all positive, including intermittent exotropia without a complicating vertical or cyclophoria component and normal random-dot stereopsis. Oculomotor skills were normal, and his visual fields were unaffected.

This patient represents one end of the continuum of ABI patients that optometrists encounter in practice. It is plausible that TM had a mild convergence insufficiency before the head injury, for which he was successfully compensating. The ABI may have caused a decompensation of this pre-existing condition precipitating his symptoms. Because all other aspects were normal, the treatment results were rapid and excellent. See Table 2 for summary.

Table 2. Pre-Vision Therapy and Post-Vision Therapy Test Results		
Case One		
Test	Pre-Vision Therapy	Post-Vision Therapy
Cover Test (D)	Ortho	Ortho
Cover Test (N)	10^Δ intermittent alternating exotropia at near (deviated 10 percent of the time)	6^Δ exophoria
Nearpoint of Convergence	15 cm break, 22 cm recovery	4 cm break, 6 cm recovery
Base in (N)	X/14/12^Δ	12/16/14^Δ
Base out (N)	X/18/12^Δ	X/35/25^Δ
Accommodative Amplitude	5D OD and OS	10D OD and OS
Binocular Accommodative Facility	8 cpm	8 cpm

Case Two
History
CS, a 6-year-old boy in kindergarten, sustained a closed-head injury in a motor vehicle accident. He was comatose for several days and suffered a focal seizure while in the hospital. He was discharged with left-sided motor control difficulties, although he was able to walk, and had sustained mild attention problems. Ophthalmological examination in the hospital revealed mydriasis, accommodative insufficiency and optic nerve pallor in the left eye. He was first seen in an optometric office 2 ½ years after the accident subsequent to receiving extensive physical and occupational therapy for his motor problems. His entering vision complaints included fatigue, loss of place and finger pointing with reading, and occasional frontal head-

aches in school. Prior neuropsychological testing revealed above average IQ and normal academic performance in all areas except reading, which was several months below his expected level.

Significant clinical findings

Unaided visual acuities were 6/6 (20/20) in each eye at distance and near. Refraction indicated +0.75D OU to 6/6 (20/20). The cover test revealed orthophoria at distance and 2^Δ exophoria at near. On the nearpoint of convergence, the break was 5 cm and the recovery 20 cm. Step vergences at 40 cm were BI $10/18/10^\Delta$ and BO $x/40/35^\Delta$. Accommodative amplitudes were 10D OD and 8.3D OS. He failed -2.00D lenses on binocular and monocular accommodative facility with the left eye. With the right eye, he was slow on both plus and minus, only clearing 4 cycles per minute. MEM retinoscopy showed +0.50D OD and +1.50D OS. Pupillary findings revealed a variable anisocoria, with the left pupil sometimes either smaller or larger than the right. This was true in both bright and dim illumination. There was no afferent pupillary defect. Confrontation fields were full, and internal and external ocular health was normal.

Diagnosis

Accommodative insufficiency (OS > OD) and increased lag of accommodation (OS only), mild convergence insufficiency, pupillary disturbance OS

Treatment

The following Rx was prescribed: OD +0.50D, OS +0.50D with a +1.00D add for the left eye only. Follow-up in six weeks revealed less fatigue and loss of place as well as better reading fluency, although some symptoms persisted. Near findings were unchanged except that the MEM was now balanced with the monocular add. In-office and home vision therapy were recommended following the treatment regimen for accommodative and convergence insufficiency of Scheiman and Wick.[24]

Outcome

The patient completed 24 sessions of therapy over 16 weeks. At the reevaluation, he was asymptomatic. He could read for short periods without his glasses, but still preferred them for extended reading and close work. All near findings were normalized except the lag of accommodation showed a +0.75D difference. Subsequently, the patient has been seen for follow-ups over a two-year period. The lag has remained the same, and he still feels more comfortable with the monocular add. His other accommodative and convergence findings have remained normal.

Factors affecting outcome

One of the prognostic factors suggested by some authors is age, and the concern is that vision therapy may be less effective in adults than children. The literature on vision therapy effectiveness suggests, however, that vision therapy can be successful across all age levels. A number of studies show excellent success in adults with binocular vision disorders. [25-27] The issue that seems to be important is cognitive/developmental level rather than age of the patient. While these abilities are related to age to some degree, we have found that patients can succeed in a vision therapy program if they have the cognitive and developmental ability typical of a 6- to 7-year-old child. In the series of cases presented here, we have demonstrated good success in adults between the ages of 19 and 49 years old.

This particular case demonstrates that vision therapy can be successful in a young child. This 6-year-old was able to complete a vision therapy program in an average period of time (12-24 visits) for a child despite the mild attention problems. Children generally require more office visits than adults,[24] and the difference in the number of sessions required by this child vs. the adult with similar problems in case one is typical of the general vision therapy population.

At the start of treatment we were concerned that the unequal accommodation amplitudes would create an obstacle to success. After prescribing an unequal add for CS, the treatment proceeded without any unusual difficulty. However, it is a factor that may complicate treatment. See Table 3 for summary.

Table 3. Pre-Vision Therapy and Post-Vision Therapy Test Results		
Case Two		
Test	Pre-Vision Therapy	Post-Vision Therapy
Cover Test (D)	Ortho	Ortho
Cover Test (N)	2^Δ exophoria	Ortho
Nearpoint of Convergence	5 cm break, 20 cm recovery	2.5 cm/7.5 cm
Base-in (N)$^\Delta$	$10/18/10^\Delta$	$X/14/12^\Delta$
Base-out (N)$^\Delta$	$X/40/35^\Delta$	$X/40/35^\Delta$
Accommodative Amplitude	10D OD and 8D OS	13D OD and OS
Binocular Accommodative Facility	0 cpm, fails –2.00D	15 cpm
Monocular Accommodative Facility	OD 4 cpm, OS 0 cpm, fails –2.00D	OD 15 cpm, OS 15 cpm
MEM Retinoscopy	OD +0.50D, OS +1.50D	OD +0.25D, O +1.00D

Case Three
History
NH, a 32-year-old white female, required surgery to remove two cerebral aneurysms. Postoperatively, she experienced mild expressive dysphasia and difficulty focusing on objects at near. She had a vision examination eight months after the surgery as the focusing problems were not improving. She was diagnosed with an accommodative insufficiency, and reading glasses were prescribed. A one-month follow-up revealed little improvement with the reading glasses, and she was referred for a vision therapy consultation.

We first examined NH 10 months after the neurosurgery. At that time she complained of an inability to focus on near tasks. She described a "weird" feeling when trying to read and developed headaches if she continued. The focusing problem was so severe that to read the newspaper she would sit on a chair and place the newspaper on the floor. NH also experienced mild cognitive and memory problems as a result of the ABI.

Significant clinical findings
Current glasses (reading only): OD +1.25D, OS +1.25D

Visual acuity (with correction) at distance and near was 6/6 (20/20) OD, OS and OU. The cover test revealed orthophoria at 20 feet and a 2^Δ comitant right hyperphoria at near. The refraction was OD -0.75D, OS -1.00D. She had 40 seconds of arc stereopsis and random-dot stereopsis. The nearpoint of convergence was receded with a break at 10 cm and a recovery at 25 cm. Step vergence ranges at near were base-in $X/18/16^\Delta$ and base-out $10/14/8^\Delta$. NH was able to complete 5 cpm with vergence facility testing (12^Δ BO/3 BI), having difficulty regaining fusion with 12^Δ base-out. The amplitude of accommodation was 3D in each eye.

Diagnosis
Convergence insufficiency, right hyperphoria, accommodative insufficiency

Treatment
The previous practitioner either did not detect or decided not to treat the hyperphoria and convergence insufficiency. We prescribed OD plano with 1^Δ BD, OS -0.25D for all near tasks and initiated a vision therapy program that followed the sequence recommended by Scheiman and Wick [24] for convergence insufficiency, accommodative insufficiency and hyperphoria.

Outcome

NH required 22 office visits to complete the vision therapy program. At the reevaluation she was asymptomatic and could now read for as long as necessary without developing either eyestrain or blur.

Factors affecting outcome

This case is similar to the first two except that a comitant vertical deviation was present. It is likely that the vertical deviation and the cognitive issues extended the therapy, hence requiring twice as many visits as the simpler convergence insufficiency presented in case one. It is important to note that this was a comitant vertical deviation without excyclotorsion, and the final outcome was excellent. Contrast the results in this instance with cases eight and nine in which excyclotorsion was present. See Table 4 for summary.

Table 4. Pre-Vision Therapy and Post-Vision Therapy Test Results		
Case Three		
Test	Pre-Vision Therapy	Post-Vision Therapy
Cover Test (D)	Orthophoria	Orthophoria
Cover Test (N)	2^Δ right hyperphoria	2^Δ right hyperphoria
Nearpoint of Convergence	10 cm break, 25 cm recovery	4 cm break, 6 cm recovery
Base in (N)	X/18/16$^\Delta$	X/18/16$^\Delta$
Base out (N)	10/14/8$^\Delta$	12/22/14$^\Delta$
Vergence Facility (12 BO/3 BI)	5 cpm	12 cpm
Accommodative Amplitude	3D OD and OS	7D OD and OS

Case Four
History

JF, a 19-year-old, sustained head trauma as a result of an automobile accident nine months prior to the examination. He was in a coma for one month and subsequently received six weeks of physical, occupational and speech therapy. He complained of difficulty focusing and concentrating when reading, trouble focusing from far to near, and very slow reading speed. He experienced eyestrain, blur and intermittent diplopia after 10 minutes of reading. While in the rehabilitation hospital, JF was examined by an optometrist who prescribed glasses with prism. These glasses did not relieve his symptoms. His goal was to improve reading comfort and speed so that he could return to college.

Significant clinical findings

Prescription: OD -1.00D with 1^Δ base-in, OS -1.00D with 1^Δ base-in. Visual acuity (with correction) at distance and near was 6/6 (20/20) OD, OS and OU. The cover test revealed orthophoria at 20 feet and a 10-12$^\Delta$ intermittent alternating exotropia at near (deviated 50 percent of the time). He had 20 seconds of arc stereopsis and random-dot stereopsis. The nearpoint of convergence was receded with a break at 20 cm and a recovery at 25 cm. Step vergence ranges at near were base-in 16/18/4$^\Delta$ and base-out X/6/-2$^\Delta$. JF was unable to complete one cycle per minute with vergence facility testing (12 BO/3 BI$^\Delta$). The amplitude of accommodation was 8D with both the right and left eyes, and he was unable to clear –2.00D lenses either binocularly or monocularly. Saccadic eye movements were evaluated using the Developmental Eye Movement Test (DEM). He scored below the first percentile in both speed and accuracy when compared to the 13-year-old level normative data. Internal and external ocular health was normal, but visual field testing revealed a right homonymous hemianopia.

Diagnosis

Convergence insufficiency, accommodative insufficiency, oculomotor dysfunction, right homonymous hemianopia

Treatment

JF was requested to read without his glasses, and a vision therapy program was recommended. The vision therapy program followed the sequence of Scheiman and Wick [24] for convergence insufficiency, accommodative insufficiency and oculomotor disorders. To help JF compensate for the right hemianopia, he was advised to rotate his book 45 to 90 degrees when reading. This compensatory strategy, suggested by Hellerstein and Fishman, [28] is designed to move the print into his normal visual field.

Outcome

JF required 32 office visits to complete the vision therapy program. At the reevaluation, JF reported elimination of all focusing problems. He could now read for as long as necessary without headaches or eyestrain. Although he was comfortable, he continued to experience difficulty with regard to his reading speed and often lost his place when reading. He reported that holding the book at an angle improved his accuracy, although his reading rate was less than desirable.

Factors affecting outcome

Although this patient sustained rather severe head trauma, he experienced only mild cognitive deficiencies. He was highly motivated to return to college where he maintained excellent mental and physical stamina as well as normal memory abilities. His attendance at therapy sessions was nearly perfect.

The characteristics of his binocular and accommodative problems were also positive. He had a small comitant intermittent exodeviation, with normal random-dot stereopsis. He also had equal accommodative abilities in each eye.

Despite these positive factors, JF only achieved partial success due to the residual saccadic fixation problems that were attributable to the right homonymous hemianopia. Although the number of errors on the DEM decreased from 30 to only four, his ratio score (speed) did not significantly improve. The reading difficulties experienced by patients with a right hemianopia may also be related to language-based problems associated with left hemispheric damage. Clearly, the presence of a hemianopia has a significant effect on outcome with vision therapy. See Table 5 for summary.

Table 5.		
Pre-Vision Therapy and Post-Vision Therapy Test Results		
Case Four		
Test	Pre-Vision Therapy	Post-Vision Therapy
Cover Test (D)	Ortho	Ortho
Cover Test (N)	10^Δ intermittent alternating exotropia at near (deviated 50 percent of the time)	$6\text{-}8^\Delta$ exophoria
Nearpoint of Convergence	20 cm break, 25 cm recovery	2 cm break, 5 cm recovery
Base in (N)	$16/18/4^\Delta$	$20/25/20^\Delta$
Base out (N)	$X/6/-2^\Delta$	$15/25/20^\Delta$
Vergence Facility (12 BO/3 BI)	0 cpm	15 cpm
Accommodative Amplitude	8D OD and OS	13D OD and OS
Binocular Accommodative Facility	0 cpm	8 cpm
Monocular Accommodative Facility	0 cpm	10 cpm
DEM Error Score	30	4
DEM Ratio Score	3.10	2.77

Case Five
History
DB, a 44-year-old school superintendent, was just about to finish his doctoral degree when he was involved in serious automobile accident. While stopped at a red light, his car was struck from behind, and he was struck in the back of his head by his briefcase, which had been on the back seat. He remembers being dazed and disoriented after the injury. Several days later he complained of headaches, neck pain, shoulder pain, left hand paresthesias, photosensitivity, blurred vision and diplopia. He was evaluated at a local rehabilitation hospital and had x-rays and a CT scan, which were negative. He received outpatient physical therapy for the head, neck and left upper extremity pain. He subsequently began experiencing problems with speech, memory, concentration, emotional lability, depression and anxiety.

We first examined him one year after his injury. DB complained that he was unable to read comfortably for even short periods of time. When he attempted to read he experienced blurred vision, diplopia and headaches. He had been examined within the past six months and was prescribed spectacles which DB felt did not help.

Significant clinical findings
Prescription: OD +0.25D, OS +0.25D, +2.25D add

Visual acuity (with correction) at distance and near was 6/18 (20/60) OD, OS and OU. We were unable to correct visual acuity to 20/20. Ocular health was normal, and there was no obvious cause of the reduced visual acuity. The cover test revealed orthophoria at 20 feet and 6-8$^\Delta$ exophoria at near. We could not elicit any stereopsis. The nearpoint of convergence was receded with a break at 20 cm and a recovery at 60 cm. Step vergence ranges at near were base-in X/10/6$^\Delta$ and base-out X/8/6$^\Delta$. JF was unable to complete one cycle per minute with vergence facility testing (12 BO/3$^\Delta$ BI). The amplitude of accommodation was less than 1D in each eye. He made so many errors and lost his place so frequently on the horizontal subtest of the Developmental Eye Movement Test that he could not complete the test.

Because of complaints about memory difficulties, we also performed a visual information processing evaluation. DB scored between the 1st and 15th percentile on all of the subtests of the Upper-Level Test of Visual Perceptual Skills (TVPS). On the Developmental Test of Visual Motor Integration (VMI), he scored at the 20th percentile.

Diagnosis

Convergence insufficiency, accommodative insufficiency, saccadic dysfunction, visual information processing dysfunction, photosensitivity

Treatment

The vision therapy program followed the sequence recommended by Scheiman and Wick [24] for convergence insufficiency, accommodative insufficiency and saccadic dysfunction. The therapy was performed with his habitual spectacle prescription. A reevaluation after 12 visits of vision therapy revealed minimal progress. The nearpoint of convergence was still receded with poor vergence ranges. There were slow and inaccurate saccades, and a reduced amplitude of accommodation was evident. We decided that the visual perceptual problems might be interfering with his ability to perform the visual efficiency therapy techniques. Therapy for visual analysis skills was initiated using the sequence suggested by Rouse and Borsting.[29] The next 12 therapy sessions were equally divided between visual analysis and visual efficiency techniques.

A reevaluation after 24 office visits again revealed minimal progress. We prescribed reading glasses with base-in prism (OD +2.75D with 1^Δ base-in and OS +2.75D with 1^Δ base-in) and continued vision therapy for 12 more visits.

Outcome

Results after 36 office visits of vision therapy were still disappointing. Minimal improvement was found in all of the areas being treated. He was, therefore, dismissed after 36 office visits. At the last reevaluation, he reported that even with the new spectacles he still experienced headaches and blur after short periods of reading.

Factors affecting outcome

The characteristics of DB's binocular and accommodative problems were positive, which suggested a relatively good outcome. However, the therapist working with DB noted frequent absences, poor carry-over from one session to another because of memory problems, frequent loss of attention and concentration, and an overall inability to exert the effort needed to succeed in a vision therapy program.

He also presented with significant visual information processing problems that, in conjunction with his other cognitive difficulties, contributed to the poor outcome. Despite the severity of the ABI in this case being less than the previous cases, the treatment outcome was poor. This is consistent with Krohel's [15] report that success cannot be reliably predicted on an individual basis from the type or severity of trauma. See Table 6 for summary.

Table 6. Pre-Vision Therapy and Post-Vision Therapy Test Results		
Case Five		
Test	Pre-Vision Therapy	Post-Vision Therapy
Cover Test (D)	Ortho	Ortho
Cover Test (N)	6-8$^\Delta$ exophoria	6-8$^\Delta$ exophoria
Nearpoint of Convergence	20 cm break, 60 cm recovery	20 cm break, 30 cm recovery
Base in (N)	X/10/6$^\Delta$	X/12/6$^\Delta$
Base out (N)	X/8/6$^\Delta$	X/10/8$^\Delta$
Vergence Facility (12 BO/3 BI)	0 cpm	0 cpm
Accommodative Amplitude	<1D OD and OS	2D OD and OS

Case Six
History

WB, a 48-year-old white male, attempted suicide with a gunshot to the left occipital lobe. Post-injury, he required neurosurgery to evacuate an intracranial hematoma. A neuro-ophthalmologist examined him four weeks after the injury and found bilateral fourth nerve palsies. A more detailed examination four months post-injury revealed anisocoria with a mild right afferent pupillary defect. Cover test indicated orthophoria at distance and near in primary gaze, 4$^\Delta$ esophoria in down gaze, 4$^\Delta$ left hyperphoria in right gaze and 2$^\Delta$ right hyperphoria in left gaze. He had underaction of both superior obliques. Visual field testing indicated a right superior quadrant defect. His accommodative amplitude was less than 1D in each eye. He was seen again by the neuro-ophthalmologist eight months post-injury. At that time, with correction (OD +1.25D-0.50X90, OS +1.25D-0.50X90, +1.50D add) his visual acuity was 6/6 (20/20) OD and OD at distance and near. He had a subtle afferent pupillary defect on the right side, but no residual bilateral fourth nerve palsies. Based on these improvements he was released from follow-up care. He had only mild cognitive deficiencies as a result of the injury.

One year later (20 months post-injury), he presented to us with significant visual complaints. He reported great frustration with reading, and he was limited to reading the large edition of Reader's Digest. His complaints included intermittent diplopia after only 10 minutes of reading, words jumping and moving around on the page, and an inability to sustain at a reading task for more than 10-15 minutes. His goal was to be able to read novels again comfortably.

Significant clinical findings
Visual acuity (with correction) at distance and near was 6/6 (20/20) OD, OS and OU. The cover test revealed orthophoria at 20 feet and at near. He had 20 seconds of arc stereopsis and random-dot stereopsis. The nearpoint of convergence was receded with a break at 12 cm and a recovery at 15 cm. Step vergence ranges at near were base-in $X/4/2^\Delta$ and base-out $x/4/2^\Delta$. WB was unable to complete one cycle per minute with vergence facility testing (12 BO/3 BI$^\Delta$). The amplitude of accommodation was 1D in each eye.

Diagnosis
Fusional vergence dysfunction, accommodative insufficiency, right superior quadrantanopia.

Treatment
The vision therapy program followed the sequence recommended by Scheiman and Wick [24] for fusional vergence dysfunction and accommodative insufficiency.

Outcome
WB required only 14 office visits to complete the vision therapy program. At the reevaluation WB reported elimination of all symptoms. He could now read for as long as necessary without eyestrain, diplopia or words appearing to move on the page. In spite of the right superior homonymous quadrantanopia, he was comfortably and quickly reading novels.

Factors affecting outcome
This patient sustained severe head trauma with only mild cognitive deficiencies. He was highly motivated to read comfortably again. The characteristics of his binocular and accommodative problems were also positive. He had only a small phoria, and his primary problems were reduced positive and negative fusional vergence ranges. Vision therapy for fusional vergence dysfunction, like convergence insufficiency, is generally very successful in the general, nonABI population.

This case demonstrates that field loss does not necessarily interfere with the final outcome of vision therapy. Although WB had a significant visual field loss, it did not affect the results of the treatment because it was a superior quadrant defect and did not affect reading. See Table 7 for summary.

Table 7. Pre-Vision Therapy and Post-Vision Therapy Test Results		
Case Six		
Test	Pre-Vision Therapy	Post-Vision Therapy
Cover Test (D)	Ortho	Ortho
Cover Test (N)	Ortho	Ortho
Nearpoint of Convergence	12 cm break, 15 cm recovery	2.5 cm break, 5 cm recovery
Base in (N)	$X/4/2^\Delta$	$X/12/10^\Delta$
Base out (N)	$X/4/2^\Delta$	$X/35/30^\Delta$
Vergence Facility (12 BO/3 BI)	0 cpm	18 cpm
Accommodative Amplitude	1D OD and OS	4D OD and OS

Case Seven
History
RF, a 61-year-old white male, was shopping in a department store when items from a shelf fell down and struck the left occipital area of his head. The item that struck him fell from a height of 6-8 feet and weighed 7 pounds. His wife reported that he was unconscious for 15 minutes. Shortly after the accident he reported a buzzing in his ears and difficulty with balance. He also reported diplopia that was present most of the time. Neurological testing revealed a mild concussion.

We examined him 18 months after the injury. At that time his primary residual complaint was diplopia. He had been to several eye doctors. The last one prescribed prism glasses to be worn at all times. RF felt that the prism glasses did not help him.

Significant clinical findings
Current glasses: OD +1.00D with 1^Δ base-down and 2^Δ base-in, OS +1.00 with 1^Δ base-up and 2^Δ base-in, +2.50D add. Visual acuity (with correction) at distance and near was 6/6 (20/20) OD, OS and OU. The cover test revealed 2-3$^\Delta$ right hyperphoria at 20 feet and 6$^\Delta$ exophoria with 2$^\Delta$ right hyperphoria at near. The deviation was comitant. The refraction was OD +1.00, OS +1.00D. He could not fuse any targets during stereopsis testing. The nearpoint of convergence revealed diplopia at all distances. Step vergence could not be measured. We used prism with the Worth 4-Dot Test to establish whether or not RF could demonstrate fusion with a second-degree target. After neutralizing the vertical misalignment, we used horizontal prism to attempt to achieve fusion. RF's responses were variable. On occasion it appeared as if he might be experiencing fusion for

brief periods of time. For the majority of time, however, RF reported that just as the images were about to fuse, they separated once again. With first-degree fusion targets in the major amblyoscope, we again found occasional fleeting fusion. The primary response, however, was inability to fuse with any combination of prism.

Diagnosis
Right hyperphoria, sensory fusion disruption syndrome

Treatment
In spite of a guarded prognosis, we prescribed a trial period of vision therapy because RF displayed fleeting fusion at times during the examination. The primary approach was to use large peripheral first- and second-degree targets. Instrumentation used included the major amblyoscope, a computer-based orthoptics program and overhead projected vectogram targets.

Outcome
No progress was noted at the reevaluation after 12 office visits. There had been no consistent progress in vision therapy. RF was unable to maintain fusion for more than a few seconds. We discontinued fusion training and presented various occlusion options to eliminate the diplopia.

Factors affecting outcome
Although there was only a small exophoria and hyperphoria which suggested a positive outcome, he was unable to maintain fusion. This presentation has been referred to as sensory fusion disruption syndrome.[30] The term refers to a condition resulting from closed-head trauma in which the patient is unable to fuse images even though they are aligned bifoveally under optimal conditions.

The prognosis in such cases is usually poor. Treatment with either lenses, prisms, vision therapy or surgery is generally unsuccessful, although there have been case reports [30,31] suggesting that some patients will regain fusion either spontaneously or with treatment. Because it is impossible to predict which cases will resolve with treatment, it is appropriate to attempt a trial period of treatment. This is another example of relatively mild head trauma with a poor final outcome. See Table 8 for summary.

Test	Pre-Vision Therapy	Post-Vision Therapy
Cover Test (D)	2-3$^\Delta$ right hyperphoria	2-3$^\Delta$ right hyperphoria
Cover Test (N)	6$^\Delta$ exophoria and 2$^\Delta$ right hyperphoria	6$^\Delta$ exophoria and 2$^\Delta$ right hyperphoria
Nearpoint of Convergence	Diplopia at all distances	Diplopia at all distances
Base in (N)	Not measurable	Not measurable
Base out (N)	Not measurable	Not measurable
Vergence Facility (12 BO/3 BI)	Not measurable	Not measurable

Table 8.
Pre-Vision Therapy and Post-Vision Therapy Test Results
Case Seven

Case Eight
History
NY, a 25-year-old female graduate student, was first seen in an acute care rehabilitation hospital about six weeks after suffering a fractured skull as a result of being struck by a car while walking. She was comatose for five days. Diplopia and nystagmus were noted upon regaining consciousness. When she was first seen in the vision clinic, she was experiencing difficulty in the following areas: memory, gait, articulation, and inappropriate affect. She was actively involved in physical, occupational, and cognitive therapy. At the time of the examination, she complained of vertical diplopia and loss of place in reading and computer activities.

Significant clinical findings
Visual acuities with a moderate myopic prescription were 6/6 (20/20) in each eye at distance and near. The cover test revealed a 4$^\Delta$ left hypertropia at distance and a 7$^\Delta$ left hypertropia at near. The left hyper increased on right gaze and left head tilt. She had a large V-pattern eso component in downgaze. Versions revealed a 2+ underacting left superior oblique and 1+ underacting right superior oblique. The Double Maddox Rod Test showed a 4-degree right excyclophoria and an 8-degree left excyclophoria. She was able to attain single vision for brief periods in left gaze with a small right head tilt. Stereopsis was absent even in that position of gaze. Monocular pursuits and saccades were normal, as were pupils, color vision, confrontation fields, and internal ocular health.

Diagnosis
Bilateral asymmetric 4th nerve palsy

Treatment

Office-based vision therapy was initiated twice a week with supplemental daily home exercises. The vision therapy involved horizontal and vertical fusional vergence training using both free-space and in-instrument techniques with an emphasis on different positions of gaze.[21] Soon after therapy commenced, we were able to prescribe 5^Δ base-down OS, which reduced her diplopia. She was able to tolerate it well enough to wear full-time. As the horizontal and vertical vergence ranges increased, the vertical diplopia decreased, but NY began complaining more about torsional diplopia. Techniques were added to improve cyclovergence, including incyclotorsion and excyclotorsion with Tranaglyphs, Eccentric Circles, afterimages and the major amblyoscope.[24]

Outcome

NY completed 45 in-office sessions over a five-month period of time, and compliance was good with 20–30 minutes of daily home therapy. At the reevaluation, she reported a significant decease in diplopia but still experienced problems in downgaze and with reading. She was very bothered by frequent torsional diplopia with small objects, which was most troublesome with reading. NY had 50 seconds of arc of random-dot stereopsis, large base-in and base-out ranges, and a small vertical vergence reserve over her prismatic glasses. Her hyper deviation in primary gaze was now equal at distance and near and reduced slightly. Interestingly, although she was able to achieve as much as 10 degrees of incyclovergence with a variety of vision therapy activities, this did not transfer to everyday activities, and her excyclophoria remained unchanged. Her range of single binocular vision was now 25–30 degrees in left, right and upgaze, but only 15 degrees in downgaze, before she experienced diplopia. The amount of prism in her glasses was reduced to 4^Δ base-down OS, and she was referred for a surgical consultation.

Surgical and post surgical treatment

A surgeon recommended bilateral torsional surgery on her superior obliques, as well as downward translation of her medial recti, to improve the V-pattern. Surgery was performed 17 months after her accident. The results showed only slight improvement in the excyclophoria, but a significant reduction in her downgaze esotropia. An additional five sessions of office-based vision therapy was performed, but again with no improvement in her torsional diplopia. Her frustration with reading led her to try an occluding contact lens because she was uncomfortable with a patch, but this was rejected after several weeks. She was able to return to college and obtained her degree during this time.

One year later, the patient was examined again after undergoing additional eye muscle surgery with a different surgeon. The torsional diplopia was again relatively unchanged, and her excyclodeviations measured 3 degrees OD and 7 degrees OS. Her vertical deviation was changed to 2^Δ right hyperphoria, and her prism was changed to 1^Δ base-down OD. She has since been lost to follow-up.

Factors affecting outcome

NY presented with only mildly impaired memory skills. She was highly motivated to eliminate the diplopia experienced when reading. Although the size of the hypertropia was small enough to manage with prisms and vision therapy, the excyclotorsion was a significant barrier. We were able to improve her horizontal and vertical fusional vergence ranges significantly. We also worked extensively on incyclotorsion, and NY was able to achieve incyclotorsion of up to 10 degrees. Despite these efforts, she continued to experience torsional diplopia when reading.

After two surgical procedures and additional postsurgical vision therapy, we were unable to eliminate the torsional diplopia. See Table 9 for summary.

Table 9. Pre-Vision Therapy and Post-Vision Therapy Test Results		
Case Eight		
Test	Pre-Vision Therapy	Post-Vision Therapy
Cover Test (D)	4^Δ left hypertropia	4^Δ left hypertropia
Cover Test (N)	7^Δ left hypertropia	4^Δ left hypertropia
Base-in (N) (with 4 base-down OS)	X/6/2$^\Delta$	X/18/14$^\Delta$
Base-out (N) (with 4 base-down OS)	X/10/4$^\Delta$	X/40/35$^\Delta$
Stereopsis (with 4 base-down OS)	None	50 seconds of arc
Double Maddox Rod Test	4° right excyclo, 8° left excyclo	4° right excyclo, 8° left excyclo
MEM Retinoscopy	OD +0.50D, OS +1.50D	OD +0.25D, OS +1.00D

Case Nine
History

LR, a 49-year-old white male, sustained a 12-foot fall from the bucket of a cherrypicker. He landed on his head and shoulder and was unconscious for five minutes. He was admitted to the hospital with a fracture to the left side of his skull and a shoulder separation. He was discharged two weeks later.

LR complained of blurred vision and intermittent diplopia and was seen by an ophthalmologist three months after the injury. He found a bilateral 4th nerve palsy with significant excyclotorsion and believed prism would not be effective because of the torsional defect. The ophthalmologist prescribed alternate occlusion and advised the patient to wait another nine months to see if the problem would resolve itself. At follow-up twelve months after the injury, LR continued to experience diplopia and difficulty reading. At that time the ophthalmologist found 2^Δ right hyperphoria in primary gaze, orthophoria in upgaze, 4^Δ right hyperphoria in right gaze with 2^Δ esophoria and 4^Δ right hyperphoria down and to the left. The Double Maddox Rod Test revealed 6 degrees of excyclotorsion of the right eye and 12 degrees of excyclotorsion of the left eye. Based on the persistent symptoms and lack of resolution, surgery was recommended. The ophthalmologist performed a right Harado-Ito procedure. At a follow-up examination four months later, the patient was ortho in right and left gaze but still had a small excyclotorsion in the right eye (4 degrees). LR was referred for a vision therapy evaluation at this time because he continued to experience eyestrain and headaches when reading.

Significant clinical findings
Current glasses: OD -2.75D-1.00x110, OS -2.75D-0.75x 80, +2.50D add.

Visual acuity (with correction) at distance and near was 6/6 (20/20) OD, OS and OU. The cover test revealed ortho at 20 feet and 2^Δ esophoria at near. Diplopia was elicited inferiorly and in lateral gaze. Double Maddox Rod testing revealed 4 degrees of excyclotorsion in the right eye. He had 60 seconds of arc stereopsis and random-dot stereopsis. The near point of convergence was slightly receded with a break at 7.5 cm and a recovery at 10 cm. Step vergence ranges at near were base-in $X/4/2^\Delta$ and base-out $X/10/6^\Delta$. LR was unable to complete one cycle per minute with vergence facility testing (12 BO/3 BI$^\Delta$).

Diagnosis
Excyclophoria, fusional vergence dysfunction

Treatment
A vision therapy program was recommended. We followed that of Scheiman and Wick [24] for fusional vergence dysfunction and cyclovertical deviations.

Outcome
LR required 16 visits of vision therapy. At the reevaluation, he reported elimination of his symptoms. His fusional vergence ranges were expanded, and he had excellent fusional facility.

Factors affecting outcome

Excyclophoria is one of the more significant negative factors influencing a successful therapeutic outcome. Vision therapy alone, in such cases, has a poor prognosis. In this case, a combination of surgery and vision therapy was successful in eliminating the patient's symptoms. See Table 10 for summary.

Table 10. Pre-Vision Therapy and Post-Vision Therapy Test Results		
Case Nine		
Test	Pre-Vision Therapy	Post-Vision Therapy
Cover Test (D)	Orthophoria	Orthophoria
Cover Test (N)	2^Δ esophoria	Orthophoria
Nearpoint of Convergence	7.5 cm and a recovery at 10 cm	4 cm and a recovery at 5 cm
Base-in (N)	X/4/2$^\Delta$	X/12/10$^\Delta$
Base-out (N)	X/10/6$^\Delta$	X/35/30$^\Delta$
Vergence Facility (12 BO/3 BI)	0 cpm, fails BI and BO$^\Delta$	10 cpm

Discussion

The treatment of binocular vision disorders associated with ABI is one of the more challenging aspects of optometric practice. Patients who survive acquired brain injury often experience multiple problems, including cognitive, psychological, motor and sensory anomalies. Even when binocular vision problems occur in isolation of cognitive and psychological issues, they are complicated. Cyclovertical and noncomitant deviations, sensory fusion anomalies, unequal accommodation, and visual field loss may accompany the basic binocular vision disorder.

Conclusions

Treatment of binocular vision disorders subsequent to ABI requires a comprehensive approach incorporating the use of lenses, prisms, occlusion, vision therapy and surgery. To make an appropriate decision about the best treatment modalities to use, it is important to understand those factors which influence the outcome. We presented a series of nine cases to demonstrate some of the important factors that should be considered when determining the prognosis for treatment of a binocular vision problem following ABI using vision therapy.

Six of the nine patients presented achieved excellent outcomes with vision therapy. The four primary factors that significantly affected our results were cognitive and perceptual problems, visual field loss, excyclotorsion and sensory fusion disruption syndrome. For example, five of the cases presented had a primary diagnosis of convergence insufficiency. Four of the five achieved good to excellent results. However, the patient with convergence insufficiency who also had cognitive, memory and attentional deficits was unable to obtain even minimal progress.

While visual field loss did not limit improvement of fusional vergence ranges, it did prevent full normalization of reading comfort and speed. In one of the cases presented, a right homonymous hemianopia continued to interfere with reading speed and comprehension even after correction of the convergence and accommodative insufficiencies. However, in another patient with a superior quadrantanopia, the outcome was excellent and the patient achieved good comfort and reading rate. The critical factor in visual field loss is whether or not it affects the functional activity in question. Since a quadrantanopia does not affect the reading task, the patient with this problem achieved an excellent outcome.

We also found that the presence of a comitant vertical deviation is not necessarily a negative factor. In such cases, prism should be used to compliment the vision therapy program, with excellent results achieved. Unfortunately, a common acquired vertical problem after head trauma is a unilateral or bilateral superior oblique palsy. This is often associated with excyclotorsion. In two of the cases presented, excyclotorsion was a significant barrier to success, although surgical treatment combined with vision therapy allowed an eventual successful outcome in one of the cases.

The final factor that interfered with outcome was the presence of sensory fusion disruption syndrome. When a patient presents with acquired diplopia after ABI, it is critical to demonstrate that fusion is present. In our experience, the ideal test to use is one that probes for random-dot stereopsis, as the presence of random-dot stereopsis is a strong positive predictor of the outcome with vision therapy.

This series of cases also support Krohel's [15] report that success cannot be reliably predicted on an individual basis from the type or severity of head trauma. In the two cases in which vision therapy results were poor, the patients sustained relatively less severe trauma than found in the other cases.

Based on these case reports, our advice is to approach the treatment of binocular vision problems associated with ABI using a multimodal sequential treatment approach. Vision therapy is an excellent option when the patient has adequate cognitive, memory and attentional skills, is able to demonstrate the presence of random-dot stereopsis, and does not have an excyclotorsional component or a hemianopia. If any of these conditions are present, vision therapy may still be appropriate, but the prognosis is guarded. We recommend a short trial period of vision therapy with follow-up to determine if additional therapy is warranted.

References

1. Cohen AH, Soden R. An optometric approach to the rehabilitation of the stroke patient. J Am Optom Assoc 1981; 52:795-800.

2. Gianutsos R. Rehabilitative optometric services for survivors of acquired brain injury. Arch Phys Med Rehabil 1988; 69:573-8.

3. Cohen AH. Optometry: the invisible member of the rehabilitation team. J Am Optom Assoc 1992; 63:529.

4. Padula WV. Editorial – An awakening. J Low Vis Neuro-Optom Rehab 1998:3-4.

5. Groffman S. Count our blessings. J Optom Vis Dev 1999; 30:43-5.

6. Cohen M, Groswasser Z, Barchadski R, Appel A. Convergence insufficiency in brain-injured patients. Brain Injury 1989;3:187-91.

7. Mitchell R, Macfarlane A, Cornell E. Ocular motility disorders following head injury. Aust Orthop J. 1983;20:31-6.

8. Suchoff IB, Kapoor N, Waxman R, Ference W. The occurrence of ocular and visual dysfunctions in an acquired brain-injured patient sample. J Am Optom Assoc 1999; 70:301-8.

9. Candler R. Some observations on orthoptic treatment following head injury. Br Orthopt J 1944;2:56-62.

10. Anderson M. Orthoptic treatment of loss of convergence and accommodation caused by road accidents ("whiplash" injury). Brit Orthopt J 1961;18:117-20.

11. Cohen AH. Visual rehabilitation of a stroke patient. J Am Optom Assoc 1978;7:831-2.

12. Soden R, Cohen AH. An optometric approach to the treatment of a non-comitant deviation. J Am Optom Assoc 1983;54:451-4.

13. Krasnow DJ. Fusional convergence loss following head trauma: a case report. Optom Monthly 1982;18-9.

14. Beck R. Ocular deviations after head injury. Am Orthopt J 1985;35:103-7.

15. Krohel GB, Kristan RW, Simon KW, Barrows N. Posttraumatic convergence insufficiency. Ann Ophthalmol 1986;18:101-4.

16. Berne SA. Visual therapy for the traumatic brain-injured. J Optom Vis Dev 1990; 21:13-6.

17. Padula WV, Shapiro JB, Jasin P. Head injury causing post trauma vision syndrome. New Eng J Optom 1988:16-21.

18. Cohen AH. Optometric management of binocular dysfunctions secondary to head trauma: case reports. J Am Optom Assoc 1992;63:569-75.

19. Hellerstein LF, Freed S. Rehabilitative optometric management of a traumatic brain injury patient. J Behav Optom 1994;5:143-8.

20. Ciuffreda KJ, Suchoff IB, Marrone MA, Ahmann E. Oculomotor rehabilitation in traumatic brain-injured patients. J Behav Optom 1996;7:31-7.

21. Flom MC. The prognosis in strabismus. Am J Optom Arch Am Acad Optom 1958;35:509-14.

22. Ludlam WM. Orthoptic treatment of strabismus. Am J Optom Arch Am Acad Optom 1961;38:369-88.

23. Caloroso EE, Rouse MW. Clinical management of strabismus. Boston: Butterworth-Heinemann, 1993.

24. Scheiman M, Wick B. Clinical management of binocular vision: heterophoric, accommodative and eye movement disorders. Philadelphia: JB Lippincott, 1994.

25. Wick B. Vision training for presbyopic nonstrabismic patients. Am J Optom Physiol Opt 1977; 54:244-7.

26. Cohen AH, Soden R. Effectiveness of visual therapy for convergence insufficiencies for an adult population. J Am Optom Assoc 1984; 55:491-4.

27. Birnbaum MH, Soden R, Cohen AH. Efficacy of vision therapy for convergence insufficiency in an adult male population. J Am Optom Assoc 1999;70:225-32.

28. Hellerstein LF, Fishman BI. Visual rehabilitation for patients with brain injury. In: Scheiman M, ed. Understanding and Managing Visual Deficits: A Guide for Occupational Therapists. Thorofare, NJ: Slack Inc, 1997.

29. Rouse MW, Borsting E. Management of visual information processing. In Scheiman M, Rouse MW, eds. Optometric Management of Learning Related Vision Problems. St. Louis: Mosby, 1994.

30. London R, Scott SH. Sensory fusion disruption syndrome. J Am Optom Assoc 1987;58:544-46.

31. Pratt-Johnson JA, Tillson G. The loss of fusion in adults with intractable diplopia (central fusion disruption). Aust New Zealand J Ophthalmol 1988;16:81-5.

An Expanded Visual Field Assessment for Brain-Injured Patients

Rosamond Gianutsos, Ph.D.
Irwin B. Suchoff, O.D., D.O.S.

Introduction

People with visual field loss associated with central nervous system injury typically report seeing more than would be expected based on their perimetrically-measured fields. Sometimes this difference is substantial, and it may or may not be associated with a neurologically-based hemi-inattention. In this chapter, the term "neglect" will be avoided because there is a lack of consensus on its definition. Rather, the theme will be on the differences between conventional objectively-determined peri- metric fields, behaviorally-determined functional fields, and patently subjective estimates of the visual fields. In brain injury rehabilitation, these differences may explain the risky, irrational behavior of some persons with visual field losses, e.g., those who continue to drive despite documented homonymous hemianopia. Lest one attribute this to a generalized cognitive decline or poor judgment caused by brain injury, those brain injury survivors with other sequelae such as intense light sensitivity or diplopia who do cease driving must be considered. On the other hand information gleaned from functionally-based visual field testing can at times explain patient behaviors that are not accounted for by conventional perimetric testing, e.g., the individual with apparently normal visual fields who continues to have left-sided car accidents when driving.

The term "metavision" [1] is used to refer to what individuals think they can see. This parallels the terms "metacognition" and "metamemory." Cognitive psychologists apply these words respectively to how people believe their minds function generally, and to what they believe they can, or will, remember. Determining the metavision of the field of vision is somewhat complex since neurologically-intact individuals are not aware of the gaps, such as those attributed to the optic nerve head, i.e., the physiological blind spot. This area, approximately the size of an orange at arm's length, is completely and abruptly devoid of sensory receptors. Nevertheless, Sergent [2] cautioned against equating the unawareness of the physiological blind spot with unawareness of neurologically-based field loss. Without making assumptions, it is important when working with brain injury survivors to evaluate both basic visual parameters and metavision.

This chapter will first briefly present an overview of conventional visual field testing that is provided to patients who have incurred acquired brain injury (ABI).[4] Then, in the interest of metavision, a subjective visual field procedure will be discussed. It is designed to go beyond usual clinical interview techniques and to yield findings that can be directly compared with the findings of conventional perimetric fields. Clinically, the subjective visual field protocol can be used with survivors of brain injury to make explicit the disparity between subjectively and objectively measured fields. Finally, several existing computer-based methods to assess an individual's visual field functioning under dynamic conditions will be presented.

Conventional Methods Of Visual Field Assessment

Confrontation field is the most common method of visual field measurement, despite its insensitivity.[3] It is performed by neurologists and rehabilitation specialists who staff acute care settings. In this method, the tester both monitors the patient's fixation and presents the stimuli. Our clinical experience with a two-person confrontation method as illustrated in Figure 1 suggests a significant improvement with regard to sensitivity.[4,5] One clinician has the singular task of monitoring the patient's fixation. The other clinician, who is behind the patient, tests for the extent of the field by introducing a moving finger in the various meridians. The same two-person method is then used to test for extinction by simultaneously presenting one or two fingers in the various quadrants of the opposite lateral hemifields. In both parts of the two-person confrontation method, there is reduced stimulus cueing. This is because the clinician presenting the fingers limits arm and body action as opposed to the one-person confrontation method.

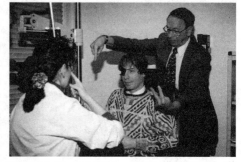

Figure 1. The two-person method offers increased sensitivity over the traditional one-person method.[4]

Tangent screen perimetry (also known as campimetry or the Bjerrum screen) is a manual visual field assessment procedure in which a wall-mounted black felt screen is used to create a map of the areas seen by a patient fixating a central point. The examiner uses a wand with a stimulus mounted on one side of the tip. The stimulus is placed at each testing point and exposed by rotating the wand. Isopters (boundaries of equivisible areas) are marked for different size stimuli. This low-tech method requires time and considerable clinical skill. It has largely been replaced in modern optometric clinics, although it is used for patients who are physically unable to be positioned for projection perimetry (see below).

The Amsler grid, shown in Figure 2, is the conventional measure of perifoveal fields. It is rarely used with survivors of central nervous system injury, because it requires a high level of concentration and cognition to fixate on one position while evaluating what is seen elsewhere.

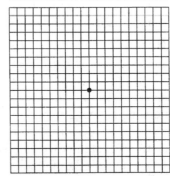

University Optometric Center
AMSLER GRID
Instructions to Patient

It is important to follow the instructions below.

1. Wear glasses, if necessary and place the grid 13 inches directly in front of area of vision.
2. Close one eye and look at the dot in the center of the grid.
3. While looking at the dot, note any interruptions, blurry areas, distorted areas or lines missing on the grid.
4. Repeat with your other eye.
5. Do this at least once a day.
6. Keep this grid in an easily accessible location.

REPORT ANY CHANGES TO YOUR EYE DOCTOR IMMEDIATELY

Figure 2. Amsler Grid

In modern optometric and ophthalmologic settings, confrontation is usually followed by projection perimetry, a procedure in which the patient is asked to fixate on an area inside a large white and diffuse hemisphere. For many years, the manual Goldmann perimeter

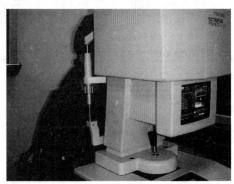

Figure 3. Perimetric assessment using the Octopus 1-2-3 perimeter.

was the standard, although others (e.g., the Tubinger perimeter) were also in use. With this type of perimeter, the clinician projects a light stimulus of varying size and brightness on preselected locations on the interior of the hemispheric test surface. Fixation is monitored through a small telescope placed on the optic nerve head—a clever technique, for if the patient is fixating properly, the scope is not visible. Most commonly, a kinetic testing approach is used, wherein the stimulus is slowly moved from the periphery towards the center, until the patient reports seeing it. Bowl perimetry permits assessment of a full 90° visual field.

Automated projection perimetric assessment, as illustrated in Figure 3, has become the standard approach. A series of brief trials is conducted using unpredictable locations and stimuli varying in intensity. Perimetric findings can offer definitive evidence of visual field loss. Although some patients are overwhelmed by the cognitive demands of the task, namely fixating while simultaneously depressing a key when an often barely visible stimulus appears, this test proves valuable.

Nonspecialists in vision do not always appreciate the important options of projection perimetry, including the scope (a full 90° is rare these days, while 30° is common) and whether each point is tested in an all-or-none, a "three zone," or a continuous (threshold) fashion. Automated perimeters differ in how they verify fixation. Certain brands use a computerized fixation monitoring technique which does not work well with some hemianopic patients. Other brands use a direct fixation monitor, which we have found to be more effective with these patients.

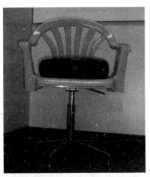

Perimetric testing is performed best when there is a sensitivity to the particular needs of the patient. Brain-injured patients most often require specialized services because of physical and cognitive limitations. Perimetric examinations require the patient to transfer into an examination chair and to sit upright for an extended period. If the perimeter can not be made wheelchair accessible, the examination chair should have arms to provide lateral trunk support as, for example, in the elevated stool adapted with an armchair top shown in Figure 4.

Figure 4. Adapted stool for making perimeters accessible to brain-injured patients

With additional time, clinical support and physical accommodation, manual or automated perimetry can usually be performed with brain-injury survivors. The examiner should appreciate the cognitive difficulty of the task, particularly that a continuous series of subtle judgments is necessary. For the patient, the ambiguity, timing and duration of this task are significant.

Perimetric methods for evaluating the perifoveal fields (central 4°) are demanding of time and attention. As with the Amsler testing method, they are frequently not used, despite the importance of the integrity of the central fields for reading and other foveated nearpoint work.

Notwithstanding the importance of optometric visual field evaluation, including perimetry, for survivors of brain injury, neither confrontation nor perimetry do much directly to promote awareness of visual field impairment. For the patient, there is a certain disconnection between the perimetric task and the perimetric testing printout, even when the examiner takes pains to explain it. Optometric visual field assessment is important for professional diagnosis. Nevertheless, in the interest of optimal care, more should be done to explain and demonstrate the impairment in a manner that is meaningful to the patient, who is often either unaware or underaware of the problem. Specifically, the visual fields need to be measured subjectively and functionally.

Subjective Visual Field Protocol

The objective is to encourage the patient to demonstrate to the examiner the apparent scope of vision in an explicit manner. Figure 5 shows a form that can be used to ask patients to sketch their own field of vision. Although this form superficially resembles the Amsler grid, experience has shown that different instructions are needed. Ordinarily, each eye is tested separately.

Instructions for subjective visual field task

1. Cover one eye.

2. Look out into the field. Notice that there are limits to the scope of what you see. For example, you do not see behind your head. Observe how far to the sides you can see without moving your eye. Do you see as far above as below, as far to the left as to the right? Try to remember what you observe.

3. Show me by drawing a chart on the paper. Blacken off areas that you do not see. Blacken off any gaps in your vision.

It is not always easy for patients to comprehend what you want them to do. Under these circumstances, it may be helpful to demonstrate that the cross-hatched circular area corresponds to the area described by one's arms forming "angel wings," as demonstrated in Figure 6. People who wear spectacles may find it helpful to consider their awareness of the rings formed by the spectacle frame. The emphasis in the instructions is to look out into the field, to judge and remember the extent of what can be seen, and then to draw this on the chart.

Although the subjective visual field protocol evolved as a formalization of a procedure used in the Head Trauma Vision Rehabilitation Unit of the

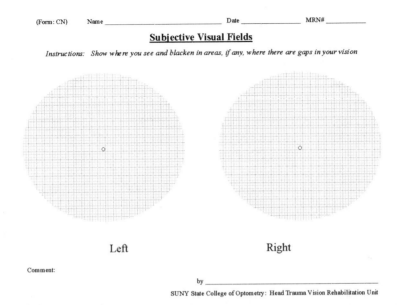

(Form: CN)   Name _____   Date _____   MRN# _____

Subjective Visual Fields

Instructions: Show where you see and blacken in areas, if any, where there are gaps in your vision

Left   Right

Comment:

by _____

SUNY State College of Optometry: Head Trauma Vision Rehabilitation Unit

Figure 5. Subjective Visual Field form.

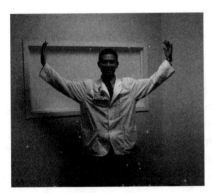

Figure 6. Angel wings demonstration for Subjective Visual Fields

State University of New York, State College of Optometry (HTVRU), it was necessary to demonstrate its feasibility with neurologically normal individuals. A sample of 25 persons was asked to sketch their visual fields according to the protocol described above. Most did not have academic training in the extent of their visual fields, although the two who did had no difficulty understanding that they were to sketch their subjective impression (not what they knew from their training).

Figure 7 shows representative drawings from the neurologically normal group. Two clear findings emerged from this normative study. First, while at the outset we were not sure if normals would report the asymmetry between the nasal and temporal fields, the drawings of most (20 out of 25) did so. Second, no subject reported a gap in the fields corresponding to the physiological blind spot. This was expected; indeed, I have used it for years to help family members and therapists understand how a person can have a gap in the field of vision and not be aware of it. As mentioned previously,

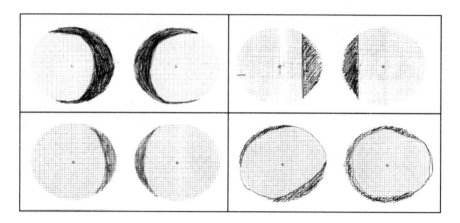

Figure 7. Subjective Visual Fields of neurologically normal individuals. These fields reflect the larger sample of 25, showing an awareness in most cases (20/25 in the sample, all but the lower right in this illustration) of the nasal temporal asymmetry of the normal fields; none shows any awareness of the physiological blind spot.

there is some dispute as to whether the lack of awareness of the physiological blind spot is the same as the unawareness of neurologically caused visual field losses,[2] and no claims are made in this regard.

The subjective visual field protocol has been used in the HTVRU for brain injury survivors with perimetrically-measured visual field loss. The results for two are shown in the top panels of Figures 8 and 9, along with their perimetric fields (lower panels). The first case example is by far the more typical, demonstrating that the subjective field underestimates the extent of perimetric loss. This patient, HW, was a 29-year-old man who had sustained head trauma and reported a variety of visual symptoms, including intermittent blurring and clearing of vision on a constant basis, difficulty making right turns when driving, and vestibular problems.

As a general rule, we have found that most brain injury survivors underestimate the perimetrically-measured loss. This finding will not surprise clinicians. The ubiquity of the term "neglect" in the neuropsychological and occupational therapy literature attests to this phenomenon. I have previously urged a more limited use of this term, to no apparent avail, and suggested alternatives such as "visual spatial hemi-imperception."[4]

The second clinical case example, BJ, is a 32-year-old man who had sustained traumatic brain injury in a fight ten years earlier, which had left him with a left homonymous hemianopia (Figure 9 bottom) and left side weakness. He has been driving safely for over five years and was employed in his profession as an engineer. BJ's subjective visual fields (Figure 9 top)

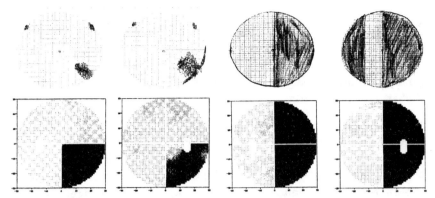

Figure 8. Subjective and perimetric visual fields of a brain injury survivor. Patient HW post-traumatic brain injury with visual-spatial hemi-inattention. Top panel shows small subjective field cuts in the lower right quadrants; the bottom panel presents the perimetric 30° threshold visual fields showing a lower right homonymous quadrantanopic defect, with it being absolute in the left eye and sparing the central 10° in the right eye.

Figure 9. Subjective and perimetric visual fields of a brain injury survivor. Patient BJ, who is 10 years post-traumatic brain injury with right homonymous hemianopia. This gentleman has been driving safely for at least 5 years. Note the congruence between his subjective (top) and his perimetric (bottom) fields. He is unusual in that he also reported an asymmetry in the intact fields.

shows the nasal-temporal asymmetry of the normal visual field. Further, his subjective fields parallel the perimetric fields.

The present approach is to advocate objective and subjective measurement of the field of vision. A further category of visual field measurement is through tasks and procedures which are practical or "functional" in nature.

Functional Visual Fields

Computerized measures of functional visual fields have been developed[4-7] for the peripheral fields: REACT (Reaction Time Measure Of Visual Fields), SDSST (Single and Double Simultaneous Stimulation), SOSH (Search for the Odd Shape), and SEARCH (Visual Search); and for the perifoveal fields: FASTREAD (Tachistoscopic Reading of Individual Words) and INSPECT (Shape Inspection). Error Detection in Texts is a useful paper and pencil procedure for perifoveal fields for persons who can read. These procedures are characterized as functional because they are practical and place fewer constraints, e.g., fixation, on the observer. The functional measures have particular value for brain injury rehabilitation because the tasks are cognitively simple. Because these procedures require nothing more than a basic personal computer, they can be conducted by therapists in rehabilitation facilities before optometric evaluations are likely to occur. These methods offer information that complements conventional optometric tests of visual fields. In addition, they can be used to promote metavision.

Peripheral Functional Visual Field Assessments

Four procedures are suggested for the peripheral fields: REACT, SDSST, SOSH, and SEARCH.

REACT takes about 2.5 minutes and requires that the observer press a response key (e.g., the primary mouse button) when a series of rapidly incrementing numbers appears anywhere on the screen. Usually, there are 5 central trials followed by 16 peripheral trials, distributed evenly in all four quadrants. When the button is pressed, the number displayed represents the response time. It is displayed briefly; then the screen clears and after a random delay the next trial begins. Depending on the distance of the observer from the screen and the size of the screen, this procedure subtends about 20°. Our recommendation is to repeat the procedure about seven times under different conditions:

1. binocular, without fixation
2. binocular, without fixation, with distraction
3. monocular, with fixation

REACT—Fixated, Normal contrast

This and subsequent data from Patient HW (brain injury from falling object)

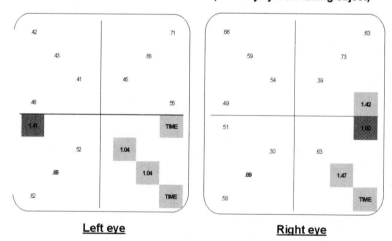

Norm = .21 sec; Clinical cutoff = .27 sec; Boldfaced = > .75 sec; Shaded = > 1.0 sec

Figure 10. REACT functional visual fields for Patient HW.

S T I M U L U S

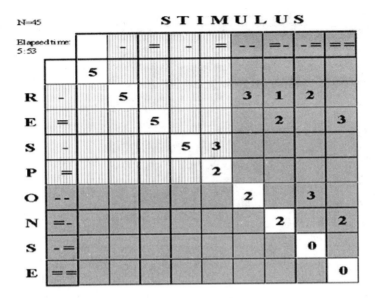

			-	=	-	=	--	=-	-=	==
Elapsed time: 5:53										
		5								
R	-		5				3	1	2	
E	=			5				2		3
S	-				5	3				
P	=					2				
O	--						2		3	
N	=-							2		2
S	-=								0	
E	==									0

Figure 11. SDSST (Single and Double Simultaneous Stimulation) results for Patient HW. The computerized SDSST involves 45 discreet trials in which all possible combinations of minus (-) and equals (=) signs are flashed for .6 sec on the far left or far right of the screen. The examiner records what the patient reports seeing. No feedback is given during the task. On this chart each column represents a given stimulus configuration and each row a particular response. Correct trials are in the main diagonal - with a maximum of 5 of each type. Normally at least 42 trials are correct. Here, the errors are excessive and involve "extinction" or reduction of the right stimulus on double trials.

4. monocular, with fixation, with reduced contrast (using 1% light transmitting NOIR filters)
5. static target (a plus sign appears, instead of the incrementing numbers).

Condition 3 most closely parallels conventional perimetry.

Not only does the observer see the briefly displayed response time, but at the end of each run there is a display of the response times in an array corresponding to where they were presented. The clinician can encourage the observer to study this display, for instance, offering a cutoff score (e.g., below .5 sec) and asking the observer to count the numbers of trials in which the cutoff was exceeded on the left and right sides respectively. This technique is designed to promote metavision. Figure 10 contains a display of REACT findings for patient HW in fixated mode. Each eye was tested separately.

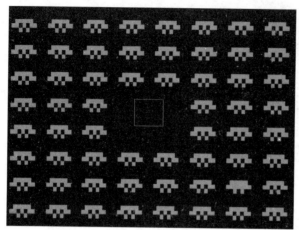

Figure 12. Stimulus display for SOSH (Search for the Odd Shape). The task is to point to the odd shape ("sleeping Martian") as quickly as possible. The examiner uses the arrow keys (or the mouse) to move the central box to the designated target. The computer saves the time from the beginning of the trial (when the "Martian falls asleep") to the when the box is first moved from the center. The trial is confirmed as correct if the box rests on the correct target. If an error is made (unlikely in SOSH), then feedback is offered and the correct target must be located. The location is retested so that reaction time results only represent correct trials.

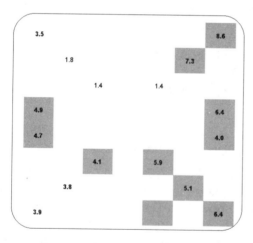

Figure 13. SOSH (Search for the Odd Shape) results for Patient HW. SOSH produces a display of reaction times (in sec) in locations corresponding to the test position. In this representation, the bold-faced times exceed 2.77 sec, or 2 standard deviations below an age-matched norm group. The shaded times exceed 3.93 sec, or 4 standard deviations below an age-matched norm group.

The remaining functional visual field tasks progressively increase the visual density and hence the attentional demands on the observer. In SDSST, the display consists of brief presentations of single or double stimuli on either the far left or far right of the computer screen. Usually, there are 45 trials representing five replications of all possible single and double displays of minus (-) and equals (=) signs. There is no fixation requirement; indeed the observer is instructed not to fixate. Figure 11 shows the SDSST results screen for HW. There is a distinct attentional component to his visual field loss, which is in addition to a perimetrically confirmed lower quadrant loss (see Figure 8). Many of his errors on SDSST involved the right side stimulus on dual presentations. For ex-

124

SEARCH: SEARCHING FOR SHAPES

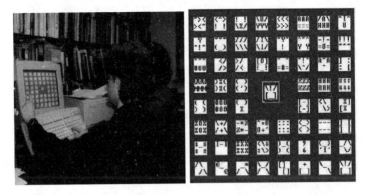

In the computerized version of SEARCH the patient points to the shape which matches the one in the center. Search time is recorded.

Figure 14. Stimulus display for SEARCH task

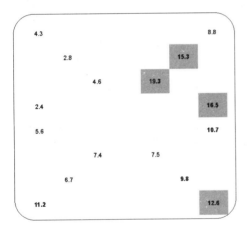

Figure 15. SEARCH (Searching for Shapes) results for Patient HW. SEARCH produces a display of reaction times (in sec) in locations corresponding to the test position. In this representation, the bold-faced times exceed the -2 standard deviation clinical cutoff of 8.94 sec. The shaded times exceed 12.60 sec, which is 4 standard deviations below an age-matched norm group.

ample, on the five trials in which he was shown two equals signs, he reported that he saw only the equals sign on the left three times. On the other two trials he thought he saw an equals sign on the left and minus on the right.

The SOSH display consists of an array, shown in Figure 12, of 60 "Martian faces." When the trial begins the observer is to find and to point to the one Martian who is "sleeping"—its "eyes" are filled in. The examiner uses the mouse or arrow keys to move the central box up to the sleeper, thereby "waking him up." The time from the display of the sleeper to the beginning of the movement of the response box from the center is captured and displayed briefly by the computer. Then the next trial begins. There are a total of 16 trials in the different locations on the screen

```
                                    FASTREAD

   DESIGNED BY:  ROSAMOND GIANUTSOS        PROGRAMMED BY:  AARON BEATTIE
     (C) 1995 LIFE SCIENCE ASSOCIATES      IBM COMPATIBLE VER #:  112295
```

SEQ	DISPLAY TIME	STIMULUS -> RESPONSE		SEQ	DISPLAY TIME	STIMULUS -> RESPONSE
1.	100	MOUSE		23.	13	ROOM
		###				####
2.	89	CRUISE		24.	11	FIELD
		###################################				####
3.	80	HAND		25.	9	ZONE
		###############################				####
4.	71	GUIDE		26.	8	READ
		############################				###
5.	63	SOUR		27.	7	READ -> READY ®
		#########################				
6.	56	LORE		28.	8	WOOD
		#######################				###
7.	50	DELAY		29.	7	BOUND
		####################				###
8.	44	BANG		30.	6	DONE
		##################				##
9.	39	PACK		31.	5	RATS
		################				##
10.	35	MOUSE		32.	4	BARK
		##############				##
11.	31	CRUSH		33.	3	NAIL -> MAID ⊘
		############				
12.	27	FIELDS -> FIELD ®		34.	4	JOIN -> JOINT ®
13.	30	TRAIN		35.	5	POOR -> POUR ⓜ
		############				
14.	26	BONG		36.	6	ROPE
		##########				##
15.	23	MAID		37.	5	REEL
		#########				##
16.	20	READ		38.	4	GUEST
		########				##
17.	17	NECK		39.	3	IDEAL -> IDEA ®
		#######				
18.	15	LORD		40.	4	BAND -> BAN ®
		######				
19.	13	ASIDE -> ASIA ®		41.	5	LORD
20.	15	LOG -> LORD ®				##
21.	17	SHOP		42.	4	DONE
		#######				##
22.	15	RED		43.	3	DELAY
		######				#
				44.	2	CHAIR -> CHAIN ®

Figure 16. A sample FASTREAD printout. (From Physical Medicine and Rehabilitation: The Complete Approach[7] with permission)

and at the end, the array of response times is shown, as in REACT. The results for patient HW (Figure 13) show excessive response times on the right side of the display, especially in the lower quadrant. As the information density increased, his functional visual field defects became more pronounced.

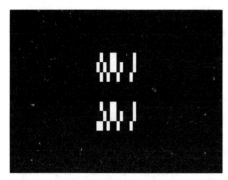

Figure 17. The INSPECT task requires that the patient indicate which side is different by pressing the left or right mouse buttons as quickly as possible.

The SEARCH task works like SOSH except that the stimuli are all different abstract patterns as shown in Figure 14. Once again, patient HW takes longer to find stimuli on the right side of the display (Figure 15).

These four peripheral functional visual field tasks progress in information density, enabling the clinician to differentiate the primary sensory loss (e.g., hemianopia) from that in

Error Detection:

- Circle every error.
- Read carefully. Do not go back over your work.
- Starting time _____   Ending time _____

Four score and seven years ago, our fathers brought forth upon this continent a new nation: conceived in liberty, and dedicated to the proposition that all men are created equal. Now we are engaged in a great civil war. . .testing whether that nation or any nation so conceived and so dedicated. . . can long endure. We are met on a great battlefield of that war.

We have come to dedicate a portion of that field as a final resting place for those who here gave their lives that this nation might live. It is altogether fitting and proper that we should do this.

But, in a larger sense, we cannot dedicate. . .we cannot consecrate. . . we cannot hallow this ground. The brave men, living and dead, who struggled here have consecrated it, far above our poor power to add or detract. The world will little note, nor long remember, what we say here, but it can never forget what they did here.

It is for us the living, rather, to be dedicated here to the unfinished work which they who fought here have thus far so nobly advanced. It is rather for us to be here dedicated to the great task remaining before us. . .that from these honored dead we take increased devotion to that cause for which they gave the last full measure of devotion. . . that we here highly resolve that these dead shall not have died in vain. . . that this nation, under God, shall have a new birth of freedom. . . and that government of the people. . .by the people. . .for the people. . . shall not perish from this earth.

Lincoln's Gettysburg Address
given November 19, 1863
on the battlefield near Gettysburg, Pennsylvania, USA

	B	E	
L	4	1	
R	5	2	FAILURES TO DETECT (out of 5/cell)

Figure 18. A sample version of Error Detection. (From Physical Medicine and Rehabilitation: The Complete Approach [7] with permission)

which there is a significant attentional component (hemi-inattention). They allow patients to experience their visual field loss and can be used to determine the extent to which they compensate for the loss. They are very practical clinically and place few performance demands on the observer apart from the visual field response. Patients can learn to perform these tasks independently, and they can be done as take-home exercises on their personal computers. In this way, patients learn how scanning and searching can be used to partially overcome the effects of the loss. In some cases, persons may improve their compensatory skills, while in most cases they discover the boundaries of compensation. This use of tasks to promote awareness is called "discovery theory" and is used productively in occupational therapy [8,9,10]

Perifoveal functional field assessments

There are three functional visual field assessment tasks for perifoveal vision. Two, FASTREAD and Error Detection in Texts, involve language, while the INSPECT program is nonverbal. The FASTREAD and INSPECT programs are computerized procedures, and Error Detection in Texts is a paper and pencil task. The verbal procedures yield much information, and so INSPECT is reserved for situations where language is an issue. At the moment these materials are standardized for English. While they could be rendered into another script-based language, they would not lend themselves to an iconic language (e.g., Chinese). For aphasics, FASTREAD and Error Detection may be useful; however, INSPECT should be used to confirm the findings nonverbally.

FASTREAD is a tachistoscopic reading task where words are flashed individually in the center of the screen of an IBM compatible computer. The individual is to say or type the word—usually the examiner types during an evaluation, unless the individual types well. If the response is correct, a prompt for the next trial is given; otherwise, the individual may be given feedback (a task option). FASTREAD begins with a 1 sec exposure which is decreased (or increased) based on the individual's performance. Typically, the trials become faster until the individual begins to make mistakes. The exposure slows until the individual once again succeeds. Performance levels off, and the "consistently best time" after 50 trials is recorded. Errors are analyzed based on whether they involve initial letters of words (L), final letters (R), or middle letters only (M). A standard list of common nouns is used for evaluation. A sample FASTREAD printout is offered in Figure 16. Many other lists are available for therapy, including words of different lengths and lists containing words where the first or last letters can be easily changed to form another word (to challenge persons who tend to misread the beginnings or endings of words).

In INSPECT, two nearly identical nonsensical shapes are displayed one above the other in the center of a computer screen as illustrated in Figure 17. There is a small difference on either the right or left side of the display. The task is to push a button on the left or right side corresponding to the location of the spatial difference. The computer records response times based on the location of the difference.

Error Detection in Texts is a paper and pencil task. There are two forms for assessment with normative information for adults. A sample version of Error Detection is shown in Figure 18. This particular example was prepared for training purposes, and it was performed by a stroke patient with a left homonymous hemianopia. Patients are to circle all spelling errors. Although time is not limited, it is recorded. They are not to go back over their work. The examiner underlines any undetected errors and classifies them based on their location (left or right side of the page) and the part of the word involved (beginning or end).

Almost any text can be used for therapy—we have developed materials which contain 24 errors on every page distributed equally into the four categories. We teach patients to record starting and ending times and later to attempt to score their own work by writing a number above each error – the goal being to find all 24 errors. Scoring helps patients begin to recognize the extent and specific pattern of their visual problem, i.e., it is a way of promoting metavision.

Conclusions

Assessment of the visual fields is particularly important for individuals who have sustained acquired brain injury. However, it is complex for a number of reasons, and as Kapoor et al.[11] have suggested, hemianopias can lie on a continuum from complete awareness to complete unawareness of the visual loss. Consequently, in the interest of optimal care in terms of more precise diagnosis that is communicated to all members of the rehabilitation team, and patient awareness of the subjective and functional implications and consequences:

- All persons who have sustained brain injury should receive a comprehensive rehabilitative optometric evaluation, especially with regard to their visual fields.
- This evaluation should include two-person confrontation and perimetric visual field assessment.
- New assessment procedures that can be part of the optometric evaluation or can be performed by allied rehabilitation clinicians include Subjective Visual Fields and Functional Visual Fields.

- The new procedures will form a bridge to rehabilitative interventions by explicitly addressing the metacognitive issue (underawareness of neurogenic visual field impairment) with Functional Visual Field assessment techniques that promote awareness.
- The central (perifoveal) visual fields should be evaluated. Further study should be made of the utility of the Amsler grid for evaluating macular sparing in brain injury survivors. The functional visual field procedures for the central fields enable us to address the practical impact of this kind of loss.

Disclosure

Dr. Gianutsos receives an authorship royalty from Life Science Associates <lifesciassoc@pipeline.com> for sales of the functional visual fields software.

References

1. Gianutsos R. Vision rehabilitation after brain injury. In: Gentile M, ed. Functional Visual Behavior: A Therapist's Guide to Evaluation and Treatment Options. Bethesda, MD: American Occupational Therapy Association, 1997:321-42.

2. Sergent J. An investigation into perceptual completion in blind areas of the visual field. Brain 1988;111:347-73.

3. Trobe JD, Acosta PC, Krischer JP, Trick GL. Confrontation visual field techniques in detection of anterior visual pathway lesions. Annals of Neurology 1981;10:28-34.

4. Gianutsos R, Suchoff IB. Visual fields after brain injury: management issues for the occupational therapist. In: Scheiman M, ed. Understanding and Managing Vision Deficits: A Guide for Occupational Therapists. Thorofare, NJ: Slack, Inc., 1997:333-58.

5. Suchoff IB, Gianutsos R, Ciuffreda KJ, Groffman S. Vision impairment related to acquired brain injury. In: Silverstone B, Lang MA, Rosenthal BP, Faye EE eds. The Lighthouse Handbook on Vision Impairment and Rehabilitation. New York: Oxford University Press, 2000:517-539.

6. Gianutsos R. Visual field deficits after brain injury: computerized screening. J Behav Optom 1991;2:143-50.

7. Suchoff IB, Gianutsos R. Rehabilitative optometric interventions for the acquired brain injured adult. In: Grabois M, Garrison SJ, Hart KA, Lemkuhl LD, eds. Physical Medicine and Rehabilitation: The Complete Approach. Cambridge, MA: Blackwell Scientific, 2000:608-21.

8. Levine DN, Calvanio R, Rinn, WE. The pathogenesis of anosognosia for hemiplegia. Neurol 1991;41:1770-81.

9. Tham K, Borell L, Gustavsson A. The discovery of disability: a phenomenological study of unilateral neglect. Am J Occup Ther 2000;54:398-406.

10. Tham K, Ginsburg E, Fisher AG, Tegner R. Training to improve awareness of disabilities in clients with unilateral neglect. Am J Occup Ther 2001;55:46-54.

11. Kapoor N, Ciuffreda KJ, Suchoff IB. Egocentric localization in patients with traumatic brain injury. In: Kapoor N, Ciuffreda KJ, Suchoff IB, eds. Visual and Vestibular Consequences of Acquired Brain Injury. Santa Ana, CA: Optometric Extension Program Foundation, 2001:131.

Egocentric Localization in Patients with Visual Neglect

Neera Kapoor, O.D., M.S.
Kenneth J. Ciuffreda, O.D., Ph.D.
Irwin B. Suchoff, O.D., D.O.S.

Introduction

While visual neglect can be one of the sequelae for stroke and traumatic brain injury, this paper will focus on neglect secondary to stroke. Of those stroke patients presenting with visual field defects, many exhibit hemianopia,[1-5] i.e., the half of the visual field contralateral to the side of the cerebral lesion loses its sensitivity to photic stimulation to varying degrees. However, there is a challenging clinical element to these field losses in that they are not always perceived by the patient.[6,7] Suchoff has characterized these hemianopic field defects from the standpoint of patient awareness, visual field testing and site of primary lesion. He conceptualizes a continuum, ranging from complete awareness (i.e., total absence of visual neglect) to complete unawareness (i.e., total visual neglect).[8] (See Figure 1.) This can account for the clinical observation that while a patient can be totally aware (or unaware) of the field loss under certain environmental, health, and/or psychological conditions, his behavior indicates total or relative unawareness (or awareness) under others. Thus, a patient who actively compensates for the hemianopia at home by scanning into the affected field may be less unaware of the loss in a more complex visual environment such as a busy street or shopping mall. The opposite can occur in the neglect patient who may become

A NO NEGLECT	B NEGLECT
⊢ —→ —→	←— ←— ⊣
1. Total awareness of field cut	1. Total unawareness of field cut
2. Favors side of field cut	2. Favors intact field
3. Hemianopia evident by conventional perimetric tests	3. Hemianopia not evident by conventional perimetric tests
4. Primary lesion in postchiasmal visual pathway	4. Primary lesion in parietal cortex

Figure 1. Continuum of hemianopic visual field. A and B are the extremes on this continuum. The arrows indicate that even when all criteria are met for the particular extreme, an individual can move to some degree toward the opposite extreme under certain environmental, health and/or psychological conditions.

131

more aware of the loss in situations where total unawareness can lead to bodily harm.

In addition to varying degrees of awareness of their visual field defect, hemianopic patients differ in their perception or sense of "straight ahead" or egocentric localization. In some patients, their subjective egocentric localization does not coincide with their objective midline representation, and thus there is a spatial mismatch between their subjective and objective visual spaces. This anomalous shift in their spatial egocenter can be 15 degrees or more with respect to the normal objective straight ahead along the body midline.[3-5,9-11] We speculate that such a mismatch between the subjective anomalous perception of straight ahead (i.e., abnormal egocentric localization) and the objective veridical straightahead (i.e., normal egocentric localization) occurs as a sequela of stroke: there is damage to the parietal lobe resulting in impaired spatial representation, especially in those patients with visual neglect (see Figure 2). Some of these patients report that they feel "un-

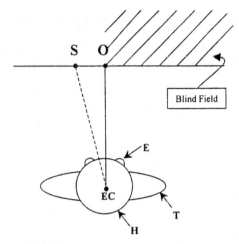

Figure 2. Schematic representation of anomalous egocentric localization in a patient with hemianopia and visual neglect (top view). Symbols: E = eyes, EC = egocenter, H = head, T = torso, O = normal objective straight-ahead, and S = anomalous subjective straight-ahead.

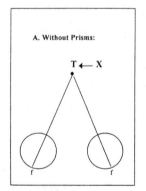 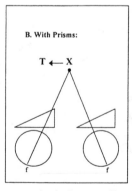

Figure 3. Schematic representation of yoked prism effect on spatial localization with the subject instructed to gaze straight ahead (top view):
A) Without the yoked prisms, where T = a midline object, X = an object to the right of midline,
B) With the yoked prisms, where objects T and X are now optically displaced laterally to the left by the prisms without any change in eye position.

steady," not "grounded," and "out of synch with the world," i.e., they manifest a disturbance in their global visual spatial sense as a result of the mismatch between veridical and their impaired perception of straight ahead. Application of yoked prism spectacles (i.e., ophthalmic prisms with their bases oriented in the same direction)[12,13] reduces the mismatch between their subjective and objective visual spaces, as the prisms optically shift the visual world in the direction of their anomalous egocentric projection with the eyes maintaining straight ahead gaze (see Figure 3). We have observed that some of these patients immediately experience greater perceptual and motor stability upon application of the yoked prisms, especially during ambulation.

Posterior Parietal Cortex Anatomy and Function

The posterior parietal cortex (PPC) is anatomically defined as the area bound posteriorly by the parieto-occipital sulcus, anteriorly by the postcentral sulcus, laterally by the posteromedial aspect of the superior temporal sulcus and the posterior part of the lateral sulcus, and medially by the subparietal sulcus.[3] Localized lesions of the PPC produce visual manifestations in stroke patients. The PPC can also incur diffuse anatomical and/or functional damage secondary to trauma, postsurgical complications, and degenerative neurological diseases (i.e., multiple sclerosis).[14]

The functions of the PPC are poorly understood. Furthermore, the specifics of the underlying mechanism related to how and why a function is executed remain uncertain.[3-5,15] However, recent research suggests that the posterior parietal area is responsible for spatial localization,[4,15-17] directing attention for voluntary oculomotor and tactile tasks,[18] and visual awareness.[3,19-21]

Recent studies[4,5,15,17,21-23] propose a multisensory model of the PPC in which it acts as a neural intermediary between the peripheral sensory inputs for the retina, muscle spindles and proprioceptive receptors complex, and the vestibular receptors, as well as their consequent motor outputs. The PPC is postulated to receive, transform and integrate the incoming sensory inputs to produce a multisensory cortical spatial representation of the world relative to the self, the environment and the object of regard.[4,17,22,23] And, lesions in this region of the right hemisphere produce classical signs and symptoms of visual neglect, such as contralesional (i.e., opposite to the side of the cerebral damage) visual inattention, impaired ability to perform visually guided tasks, and poor spatial localization and awareness. However, one important associated factor rarely explicitly expressed by patients is a shift in their subjective perception of straight ahead, or a shift in "egocentric space." That is, there is an actual shift in their perceived egocenter relative to that normally found within two degrees of one's objective midline.[4] The concept of the "egocenter" and its role in spatial localization has been well described in the literature.[2,4,15-17,22-26]

For example, Karnath[4] suggested that disruption of this egocentric, spatial representative process at any of its three proposed cortical stages (i.e., reception, transformation, and integration of the peripheral sensory information) is an essential aspect in the phenomenon of visual neglect. Further, in a patient with a lesion of the right PPC, he found a disruption in the coordinate transformation with a systematic bias or error producing an ipsilesional (i.e., the same side as the cerebral damage) shift in the patient's subjective spatial frame of reference. In close association with this anomalous spatial representation was the patient's disturbed perception of body orientation and localization within the environment. Therefore, an ipsilesional shift in a patient's spatial frame of reference, and consequently the patient's perceived global body orientation and localization, will result in an ispilesional shift in the patient's subjective sense or perception of "straight ahead" (egocentric localization) relative to the objective or veridical "straight ahead." [2,4,26]

Karnath's Experiment on Egocentric Localization and Visual Neglect

In 1994, Karnath investigated the effects of light and dark environment, proprioceptive stimulation, and vestibular (i.e., caloric) stimulation on egocentric localization in patients with visual neglect. He used an opaque, light bulb-shaped, full-body enclosure to measure egocentric localization in three patients with right brain damage, four patients with left brain damage, and ten non-brain-damaged patients who served as controls. While the patients with right brain damage manifested marked visual neglect as determined by standard line bisection and cancellation tests, there was no evidence of visual neglect in either the other patients or controls.

In each of the three visual neglect patients with right parietal lesions, there was an average 15 degree ipsilesional shift in their horizontal egocentric localization (to the right), with no manifest shift vertically. For the control group (n=14), however, there was no significant shift in egocentric localization (i.e., it was within an average of two degrees of veridical straight ahead) both horizontally and vertically, as expected in non-brain-injured individuals. Measures of egocentric localization were also compared in the dark and light environments with no significant difference noted for either the experimental or control group. This comparison was performed to ascertain the effect of environmental perceptual cues and visual feedback on subjective visual space.

Karnath also investigated the role of proprioception and the vestibular system in these same patients with left neglect. He observed a reduction of the anomalous 15 degree ipsilesional shift in egocentric localization for the neglect subjects when vibration of the left posterior neck muscles was introduced, as well as with caloric stimulation of the left external auditory canal, with each being performed separately. He noted a further reduction in the anomalous egocentric shift when the left caloric and left proprioceptive stimuli were combined. The effects of left caloric and right proprioceptive stimuli negated each other upon combination to produce no significant change in the anomalous 15 degree ipsilesional egocentric shift.

The above results confirmed the notion that patients with left visual neglect have a displaced perception of "straight ahead," with it being biased ipsilesionally. Further, the disparity between subjective and veridical straight ahead could be compensated by contralateral neck muscle proprioceptive and contralateral caloric stimulation. Such results clearly support the hypothesis of the PPC functioning as a multisensory integrator in which various peripheral afferent sources (i.e., retina, neck muscle spindles, and cupulae) contribute to one's representation of visual space.

Karnath's Experiments on Spatial Exploration

In a more recent experiment, Karnath et al.[5] measured gaze, head and eye-in-head positions, as well as the percentage of exploration time in each position across space, for a visual spatial exploration task in four patients with left neglect. These were compared with controls consisting of four right brain-damaged patients without neglect and six non-brain-damaged normal patients. The experimenters modified the interior of their bulb-shaped enclosure, as described earlier, to be covered by 340 letters, each being 2 degrees in vertical extent. The array of letters subtended a visual angle of 280 degrees horizontally (140 degrees to the right and left of the subject's midline) and 100 degrees vertically (50 degrees above and below the eye level of the subject). Each subject was seated upright in an armchair. The head was able to move freely, but the rest of the body was immobilized by shoulder straps and belts. Subjects wore a three-dimensional search coil eye movement system. In addition, a second three-dimensional coil system was mounted on the subject's forehead. These two devices objectively measured gaze and head position simultaneously. Eye-in-head position was calculated as being the difference between gaze and head positions. Subjects were instructed to search for a particular letter in the 340 letter array over 20 second intervals. During each search interval, however, the subjects were not informed that the letter for which they were instructed to search did not actually exist in the array.

In the controls, the distributions of the percentage of visual spatial exploration search time for gaze, head and eye-in-head positions were centered around the midline, with equal exploration time to the left and right. In contrast, for patients with left neglect, distributions of the percentage of search time for visual spatial exploration for gaze, head and eye-in-head positions were shifted to the same side of the lesion (to the right), with restricted extents both leftward as well as to the extreme right. The distribution centered around a point in ipsilesional space, with restricted extents both ipsilesionally and contralesionally. This was similar to that observed by Karnath et al. for the tactile domain in neglect patients.[21] However, this was contrary to Kinsbourne's model[19,20] of a lateral gradient of ipsilesional attentional orienting in neglect patients, which would predict an increase rather than the decrease observed by Karnath et al. in search times extending into extreme ipsilesional space.

Experiments on Yoked Prism Adaptation

In 1972, Welch and Goldstein[27] examined short-term adaptation to yoked prism application in brain-damaged patients, psychiatric patients (who had not incurred a stroke or head trauma), and normal adults. They used 20^Δ bases-right yoked prisms and measured the subject's accuracy of target pointing before, during and after exposure to the yoked prisms. The pre-exposure period consisted of several pointing trials in which the subject received visual feedback regarding the accuracy of pointing. This was followed by 10 pointing trials without visual feedback, where only kinesthetic information was available. Although the exposure period was not timed, it did consist of 30 target pointing trials with visual feedback, in which the subjects were informed of their errors and told to attempt to correct for these inaccuracies. Although they did not control for the hemisphere or precise location of the brain damage in the postexposure measures, Welch and Goldstein found that the brain-damaged group adapted to the yoked prisms significantly less than either the psychiatric or normal groups. That is, there was considerably less reduction in their pointing errors following the exposure period than in the other groups. This is consistent with the other studies demonstrating reduced adaptative ability in patients with brain damage.[27-29]

In 1990, Rossi et al.[28] investigated the use of 15^Δ yoked half-Fresnel prisms (i.e., prisms covering the affected hemifield of the lens only) in stroke patients with hemianopia and/or visual neglect. Standard neurologic tests (Modified Mini Mental Status Examination, Motor Free Visual Perceptual Test, Line Bisection Test, Line Cancellation Test, and Barthel ADL-Mobility Score) were performed at baseline, two weeks post-prism wear, and four weeks post-prism wear. Both sessions of post-prism testing were performed with the patients wearing the yoked prisms. Twenty-one stroke patients were assigned to the control group (i.e., no yoked prisms) and eighteen were assigned to the experimental group (i.e., Fresnel yoked prisms). Those assigned to the experimental group wore the yoked prisms for all daytime activities for the entire four weeks. Both groups received standard physical, occupational and speech rehabilitation, as well as retraining for activities of daily living (ADL) and visual perceptual tasks during this period. Those in the experimental group improved relative to the control group for the perceptual tests but not the ADL test. Further, Rossi et al. noted that the visual neglect patients within the experimental group performed consistently better than those manifesting hemianopia without neglect.

Ciuffreda et al.[9] designed a full-body, box-like enclosure enabling measurements of egocentric localization to study short-term adaptation to yoked prisms in normal young adults. Ten visually normal adult subjects wore 20^Δ bases-right yoked prisms for one hour, during which time various gross and fine motor tasks were performed continuously to enhance perceptual-motor adaptation. Horizontal egocentric localization was measured before, during and immediately after the one-hour adaptation period. A questionnaire was also used to assess perceived changes in visuoperceptual and motor control. Baseline measurements of egocentric localization prior to the application of the yoked prisms were within two degrees of the midline, which is consistent with Karnath's findings in normal individuals.[4] Measurements obtained upon initial application of the yoked prisms showed the predicted amount of optical displacement, whereas immediately after the one-hour adaptation period, there was a mean adaptation of 33% to the yoked prisms (that is, the initial effect was reduced by one-third). This concurs with the results of other studies involving sensory and motor adaptation to ophthalmic prisms.[30] More specifically, these findings regarding yoked prisms suggest that visual and postural stability can be restored, at least partially, for visually normal adults wearing yoked prisms through perceptual and motor adaptation.[10,13,14] Ongoing studies in Ciuffreda's laboratory show similar findings for vertical yoked prisms, as well as a range (5 to 20 prism diopters) of horizontal yoked prisms.

Yoked prisms have also been reported to alter body posture rapidly in patients with ABI.[13,14] Padula[13] observed that, in addition to purely visual symptoms, some ABI patients manifest abnormal posture, wherein the body's center of mass is shifted ipsilesionally. In such cases, Padula reported that the application of yoked prisms with the bases oriented contralesionally corrected the abnormal posture that was initially evident in these patients. This observation led to the speculation of a "visual midline shift syndrome" in which there is an ipsilesional shift in both the visual perception of midline and the body's center of mass.

In 1997, Gizzi et al.[14] used dynamic platform posturography to investigate the effects of yoked prisms on postural changes in normal individuals with no history of neurological, visual or vestibular disease. Dynamic platform posturography was measured pre-prism, immediately upon the application of 15^Δ bases-right yoked prisms, and one hour post-prism. During the prism exposure, the subjects ambulated freely in the outpatient hospital environment. Results revealed a small (approximately 0.30 degree) rightward shift in the subjects' mean center of gravity immediately following prism application. This shift in mean center of gravity increased from 0.30 to 1.0 degree with one hour of prism wear. Although the shift of one degree is small (the body can withstand up to ten degrees of a lateral shift without falling over), it was statistically significant. The initial post-prism findings clearly illustrate an almost immediate spatial rearrangement which was further altered after one hour of sensorimotor activity with prism wear. Another interesting point is that this spatial rearrangement became "internalized" within minutes, since posturography measurements with the eyes open and subsequently with the eyes closed were similar. Continued efforts investigating changes in the center of gravity induced by yoked prism wear for extended periods (i.e., several months) using different magnitudes of yoked prisms would add a dynamic temporal domain to these adaptation studies.

More recently, Rossetti et al.,[10] investigated short-term adaptation to yoked prisms in patients with right brain damage using midline pointing accuracy and performance on a variety of neuropsychological tests (i.e., line bisection, line cancellation, copying a drawing, drawing a daisy from memory, and reading simple text) as the basic measures. Their study involved randomly assigning patients either to a control group, who wore goggles without prism, or to an experimental group, who wore goggles containing 10^Δ bases-left yoked prisms for two hours. Midline pointing accuracy and performance on the neuropsychological tests were compared pre- and post-goggle exposure. Testing was performed with the goggles removed. The experimental group demonstrated improvement in midline pointing accuracy, as well as the neuropsychological tests, as compared with the control group. These results suggested that after only two hours of wearing yoked prisms, a true adaptive neurological change occurred at the level of egocentric spatial representation, at least partially restoring the coordinate transformation to correspond to the true objective placement of objects in space relative to the self and the environment. This striking finding should be confirmed in a larger and more diverse group of patients, as the therapeutic and neurological implications are considerable.

A New Device for Assessing Yoked Prism Adaptation and Egocentric Localization

Researchers have designed devices to measure egocentric localization in the laboratory.[4,9] While these devices have produced repeatable and reliable data from normal subjects, as well as from selected patients with head trauma-related neurological dysfunction, they have been quite large and cumbersome. Furthermore, these laboratory devices required the individual to be placed within a full-body enclosure. Thus, they are less than ideal for routine clinical practice and investigation. Therefore, we designed a small portable device using a folded optical system to circumvent the above problems with minimal complexity for use in the clinic. [10]

Our egocentric localization device is based around a 12-inch light-tight cubical enclosure. The enclosure houses a small He-Ne laser, neutral density filter, two rotatable mirrors, and two adjustable rods about which the mirrors can rotate either horizontally or vertically (see Figure 4). We tested this device on 14 visually normal, non-brain-injured individuals ranging from 23 to 53 years of age. Ten measures of egocentric localization were taken for each subject in both the horizontal and vertical directions. Subjects were instructed to keep their heads and bodies stationary and straight ahead and then to gaze straight ahead (i.e., "as if they were looking at their own eyes in a mirror reflection of themselves") without attempting to track or look directly at the laser target. Measures to the left of and below the objective midline were assigned minus values, and those to the right and above were specified as positive. The group mean, +/- 1 standard error of measurement (SEM), horizontal and vertical egocentric localization values were -0.51 +/- 1.08 deg and -0.83 +/- 0.84 deg, respectively. Individual subjects' mean, +/- 1 SEM, horizontal and vertical values ranged from -2.63 to +1.66 deg and -1.77 to +0.86 deg, respectively. These values are in agreement with the established normative data using larger and more complex laboratory devices.[4,9]

We are collecting preliminary data on brain-injured patients before yoked prism application, upon initial yoked prism application, one week post-prism application, and one month post-prism application. We hope that analysis of egocentric localization data over both short- and long-term periods will assist in providing a scientific basis for yoked prism spectacle prescription in specific categories of brain-injured patients.

Ten patients have been tested using the same instructional set for non-brain-injured persons with our new and portable egocentric localization device (see Table 1). For subjects #1 and #2, the egocentric shifts were relatively small (1.7 deg R and 3.6 deg L, respectively). The shift for subject #1 was just outside normal limits; therefore, no prisms were prescribed. There was extreme variability in subject #2's responses due to difficulty maintaining fixation. Therefore, no yoked prisms were prescribed. In seven of the eight subjects prescribed yoked prism, the results were encouraging and helped the patients' spatial abilities. Data for all subjects are shown in Table 1. The pa-

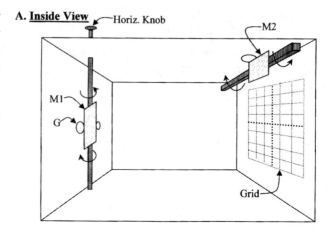

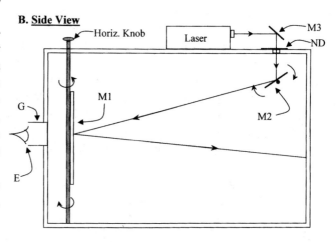

Figure 4. Egocentric localization device. A. Internal perspective view showing the viewing goggles (G), horizontally (M1) and vertically (M2) deflecting mirrors, as well as the external calibrated grid (Grid) which is visible only to the experimenters and not to the subject. B. Internal side view showing subject's eye (E), viewing goggles (G), horizontally deflecting mirror (M1), laser (top of enclosure), mirror deflecting laser target into the enclosure (M3), neutral density filter (ND), and the vertically deflecting mirror (M2).

tients' subjective responses to the yoked prism application are indicated in parentheses in Table 1 by the negative sign (subject did not respond well to the prism) and plus sign (subject reported positive subjective changes with the prisms).

Table 1.
Preliminary Data for Egocentric Localization and Yoked Prisms in Patients

Subject #	Pre-Prism	Post-Prism	One Month Later	Three Months Later
1	1.7 deg R	1.5 deg R (3.5BL)	No prism prescribed	No prism prescribed
2*	3.6 deg L	3.6 deg L (7BR)	No prism prescribed	No prism prescribed
3	7.9 deg R	9.7 deg R (7BL) (+)	8.9 deg R (+)	9.0 deg R (+)
4*	3.4 deg L	3.2 deg L (5BR) (+)	3.0 deg L (+)	3.2 deg L (+)
5*	2.9 deg L	2.3 deg L (4BR) (-)	NA (-)	NA (-)
6*	4.7 deg L	1.7 deg L (4BR) (+)	1.5 deg L (+)	1.7 deg L (+)
7	3.2 deg R	2.5 deg R (3.5BL) (+)	2.6 deg R (+)	2.4 deg R (+)
8	5.0 deg R	3.5 deg R (5 BL) (+)	3.5 deg R (+)	3.2 deg R (+)
9	4.7 deg R	2.3 deg R (4BL) (+)	2.3 deg R (+)	2.0 deg R (+)
10	3.2 deg R	2.3 deg R (3.5BL) (+)	2.5 deg R (+)	2.5 deg R (+)

*Key to symbols: *=left brain-injured patients, R=right, L=left, B=base, + = positive response to prism, and - = negative response to prism.*

These initial encouraging findings motivated us to plan future investigations of the short- and long-term effects of yoked prisms with respect to egocentric localization. Further, these results are consistent with our hypotheses regarding the use of yoked prisms as a long-term spatial rehabilitative aid in ABI patients with an abnormally shifted egocenter. We are continuing to collect preliminary data on possible long-term adaptive effects in our subjects using our new device with the current protocol.

Our current device is markedly improved as compared to the larger fully-enclosed devices with respect to clinical utility. However, there are still refinements to be made based on our experience with it thus far. First, a small infrared video camera will be installed atop the enclosure to view the patient's eye position continually. This will ensure that appropriate eye position and stability are maintained throughout the testing, as there is a natural tendency by some to gaze periodically at the moving target, which would invalidate the measurement. Second, movement of the laser target will be computer-controlled via an externally mounted x-y mirror galvanometer system. This will assure constancy of target velocity, as well as provide us with the ability to alter target velocity if needed, perhaps to find a subject's optimal performance value. Third, data acquisition and analysis will be performed by the same computer via analog-to-digital (A/D) technology and specialized software, respectively. Lastly, a head/chin rest assembly will be incorporated as an integral part of the device. This will assure both head position and stability, as well as prevent fatigue effects of the subjects during sustained head maintenance in the viewing goggles.

Future Directions

The area of stroke and visuospatial perception is fascinating. Future endeavors will involve investigating the:

1. long-term sensorimotor adaptation in hemianopic stroke patients as a function of time (up to three years) and magnitude (up to 15^Δ) of yoked prism wear using neurophysiological imaging techniques (i.e., functional MRI) to localize sites of cerebral involvement;

2. long-term sensorimotor adaptation in hemianopic stroke patients as a function of time (up to three years) and magnitude (up to 15^Δ) yoked prism wear using dynamic posturography and egocentric localization to note changes in the center of gravity and egocenter adaptation over time;

3. ability of hemianopic stroke patients to readapt their visuospatial representation upon the removal of the yoked prisms after having worn them

for varying periods (i.e., minutes, hours, days and weeks) using egocentric localization as the primary measure.

References

1. Suchoff IB, Kapoor N, Waxman R, Ference W. The occurrence of visual and ocular conditions in a non-selected acquired brain-injured patient sample. J Am Optom Assoc 1999;70:301-8.

2. Ventre J, Flandrin JM, Jeannerod M. In search for the egocentric reference. A neuropsychological hypothesis. Neuropsychologia 1984; 22:797-806.

3. Stein JF. Representation of egocentric space in the posterior parietal cortex. Quarterly J Exp Physiol 1989;74:583-606.

4. Karnath HO. Subjective body orientation in neglect and the interactive contribution of neck muscle proprioception and vestibular stimulation. Brain 1994; 117:1001-12.

5. Karnath HO, Niemeier M, Dichgans J. Space exploration in neglect. Brain1998; 121:2357-67.

6. Gianutsos R, Suchoff IB. Visual fields after brain injury: management issues for the occupational therapist. In: Scheiman M, ed. Understanding and Managing Vision Deficits: A Guide for Occupational Therapists. Thorofare, NJ: Slack, 1998.

7. Gianutsos R, Matheson P. The rehabilitation of visual perceptual disorders attributable to brain injury. In: Meier MJ, Benton AL, Diller L, eds. Neuropsychological Rehabilitation. New York: Churchill Livingstone, 1987: 202-41.

8. Suchoff IB. Lecture notes from Optometric Interventions in Acquired Brain Injury course given to residents. State University of New York, State College of Optometry, 1998.

9. Ciuffreda KJ, Kim J, Tam M, Suchoff IB. Short-term adaptation to yoked prisms. Am. Acad. Optom. poster presentation, Orlando, FL, 1996.

10. Rossetti Y, Rode G, Pisella L, Farne A, Li L, Boisson D, Perenin MT. Prism adaptation to a rightward optical deviation rehabilitates left hemispatial neglect. Nature 1998; 395:166-9.

11. Kapoor N, Ciuffreda KJ, Harris G, Suchoff IB, Kim J, Huang M, Bae P. A new portable clinical device for measuring egocentric localization. ARVO poster presentation, Fort Lauderdale, FL, 1999.

12. Zost MG. Diagnosis and management of visual dysfunction in cerebral injury. In: Maino DM, ed. Diagnosis and Management of Special Populations. St. Louis: Mosby Yearbook, 1995.

13. Padula W. Neuro-optometric Rehabilitation. Santa Ana, CA: Optometric Extension Program, 1996.

14. Gizzi M, Khattar V, Eckert A. A quantitative study of postural shifts induced by yoked prisms. J Optom Vis Dev 1997; 28: 200-3.

15. Andersen RA. Multimodal integration for the representation of space in the posterior parietal cortex. Philos Trans R Soc (Lond) B Biol Sci 1997; 352:1421-8.

16. Snyder LH, Batista A., Andersen RA. Coding of intention in the posterior parietal cortex. Nature 1993; 386:167-70.

17. Andersen RA, Snyder LH, Li C-S, Stricanne B. Coordinate transformations in the representation of spatial information. Curr Opin Neurobiol 1993; 3:171-6.

18. Crick F. Function of the thalamic reticular complex: the searchlight hypothesis. Proceedings of the National Academy of Sciences of the U.S.A. 1984;81:4586-90.

19. Kinsbourne M. Hemi-neglect and hemisphere rivalry. Adv Neurol 1977;18: 41-9.

20. Kinsbourne M. Mechanisms of unilateral neglect. In: Jeannerod M, ed. Neurophysiological and Neuropsychological Aspects of Spatial Neglect. Amsterdam, North-Holland: Elsevier, 1987.

21. Karnath HO, Perenin MT. Tactile exploration of peripersonal space in patients with neglect. Neuroreport 1998; 9:2273-7.

22. Mennemeier M, Chatterjee A, Heilman KM. A comparison of the influences of body and environment centered reference frames on neglect. Brain 1994;117:1013-21.

23. Snyder LH, Grieve K., Brotchie P, Andersen RA. Separate body-and world-referenced representations of visual space in parietal cortex. Nature 1998;394:887-90.

24. Head H. Studies in Neurology. Oxford: Oxford University Press, 1920.

25. Bisiach E, Capitani E, Porta E. Two basic properties of space representation in the brain: evidence from unilateral neglect. J Neurol Neurosurg Psychiatry 1985; 48:141-4.

26. Biguer B, Donaldson IML, Hein A, Jeannerod M. Neck muscle vibration modifies the representation of visual motion and direction in man. Brain 1988;111:1405-24.

27. Welch RB, Goldstein G. Prism adaptation and brain damage. Neuropsychologia 1972; 10:387-94.

28. Rossi PW, Kheyfets S, Reding MJ. Fresnel prisms improve visual perception in stroke patients with homonymous hemianopia or unilateral visual neglect. Neurology 1990; 40:1597-9.

29. Diller L, Weinberg J. Hemi-inattention and rehabilitation: the evolution of a rational treatment program. In: Weinstein EA, Freidland RP, eds. Advances in Neurology (Vol. 18) New York: Raven Press, 1977.

30. Welch RB Perceptual Modification. New York: Academic Press, 1978:13-106.

Altered Visual Adaptation in Patients with Traumatic Brain Injury

Mary M. Jackowski, Ph.D., O.D.

Introduction

Traumatic brain injury (TBI) is an insult to the brain, not of degenerative or congenital nature, but one caused by an external force that can produce impairments of cognitive ability or physical functioning. The 1991 National Health Interview Survey identified the yearly incidence of mild to moderate TBI to be 618 per 100,000 persons.[1] Approximately 370,000 Americans are hospitalized annually as a result of TBI; 99,000 sustain moderate to severe brain injuries resulting in chronic disabling conditions,[2] while TBI claims more than 56,000 lives each year.[3] Annual direct medical costs of TBI in the United States are estimated at 48.3 billion dollars.[4]

Advances in medical technology have increased the number of individuals surviving TBI, thus producing the socioeconomic consequences of a growing number of persons with disabilities. Of the various functional deficits demonstrated, chronic visual dysfunction is often profoundly disabling for patients returning to work and daily living activities. TBI patients can exhibit various visual deficits, including accommodative, binocular and/or oculomotor dysfunction, altered refractive error, visual field loss and perceptual deficits.[5-10] TBI can be associated with ocular damage and/or postretinal injury of the visual pathways. However, even mild TBI associated with whiplash or cervical strain can cause visual disability, often without clear evidence of ocular or cerebral damage. Padula has identified the collection of visual signs and symptoms resulting from TBI as Post-Trauma Vision Syndrome (PTVS). These may include asthenopia, headache, diplopia, focusing inability, and difficulty with fixation and tracking.[11] Reports of strabismus, convergence insufficiency, divergence excess, and accommodative insufficiency have been cited in the literature for many years. Gianutsos et al.[12] have reported the high prevalence of reduced visual acuity, deficient accommodation, and complaints of diplopia among survivors of traumatic brain injury; exophoria and exotropia are commonly identified within this same population. Optometric management of these visual deficits, including standard objective measures and visual treatment

145

modalities, has been successful in alleviating much of the visual discomfort associated with TBI. However, more elusive yet commonly reported symptoms associated with ambient illumination (including atypical light sensitivity, photic-driven headache, and reduced or prolonged dark adaptation[13-15]) have received far less attention, despite their often profoundly disabling effects.

Because there is often litigation when personal injuries are involved, especially when complaints persist, the validity of disabling symptoms that extend beyond the first few months of recovery is often called into question. Our purpose here is to review recent reports and preliminary data from our laboratories and those of other investigators who have focused on the objective measurements of alterations in visual adaptation following TBI and the quantitative assessment of available treatment regimens.

Light sensitivity

Patients who have sustained traumatic brain injury often experience a new, intense and chronic light sensitivity, severe enough to encumber their rehabilitation and return to daily work and recreation. In one study, 44% of patients with TBI spontaneously complained of discomfort in bright illumination; even greater numbers displayed a lowered threshold for luminance tolerance,[16] thus suggesting the significant underreporting of light sensitivity in this population. Light sensitivity is broadly defined as an intolerance to light, an incompletely understood subjective symptom, having both ocular and non-ocular origins. Although ocular damage can occur in brain injury, many subjects with TBI-induced photosensitivity have good ocular health. This non-ocular photosensitivity is noted in a variety of neurologic disorders such as meningitis, thalamic infarcts, trigeminal neuralgia, migraine, subarachnoid hemorrhage, cerebral hypoxia, tumors of the anterior pathway, and mild to severe brain injuries.[14,17]

Few studies specifically address the intolerance to high levels of light that can be exhibited in the post-traumatic period. Of these, reports of persistent light sensitivity after brain injury have focused on the first few weeks or months past injury.[18] One study by Bohnen et al.[19] documented the use of psychophysical methods to quantify a significant light sensitivity in post-concussional subjects six months after mild brain injury. Our clinical experience with light-sensitive patients following TBI has been remarkable for the consistent and often surprising results provided by use of short wavelength light-filtering lenses. These lenses have been used with dramatic success for many years in the treatment of light sensitivity and glare sensitivity in patients with significant ocular disease(s); treatment of patients with light sensitivity of non-ocular origin was a natural extension of the use of these lenses, despite the absence of any clear mechanism of action. Since little quantification of vision enhancement or actual functional testing had been reported concerning these filters, our initial goal was to identify simple clinical methods to measure effects of these and other light-filtering lenses on the visual function of patients who report TBI-induced light sensitivity, especially in those patients who have complaints beyond the first few months post-injury. By matching patients' descriptions of altered visual perception (reduced image clarity/contrast, decreased reading comfort, etc.) with measures of visual performance (contrast sensitivity and reading rate), data were collected that provided objective evidence for improvement of visual function using specific light-filtering lenses.

Methods
Subjects
Seven control subjects, three men and four women, ranging in age from 24 to 48 years, were selected at random from the staff of the SUNY, Syracuse, Department of Ophthalmology and their family members. Control subjects had no previous history of TBI and denied any learning or reading disability. Each subject had graduated from high school; four had college education. All had received a complete ocular and visual examination within six months of testing. They had no history of amblyopia or any eye disease that might affect vision, were not medically treated for diabetes mellitus, did not use medications toxic to ocular structures, nor had a refractive error of >6D of sphere or >3D of cylinder. All subjects exhibited normal ocular health and were corrected to 20/20 at both distance and near prior to testing.

Seven experimental subjects were identified through optometric examinations conducted on patients who had experienced traumatic brain injury. Three men and four women ranging in age from 29 to 42 years were tested. No patient reported pre-morbid learning disability or reading difficulty. Patients conformed to the exclusion criteria set for the control group (one exception was DB; the presence of a small off-axis corneal scar and modest nuclear lens changes were considered visually insignificant). Tables 1a and 1b provide descriptions of the seven subjects who reported light sensitivity and difficulty with reading as a result of brain injury. This is a highly heterogeneous population in terms of visual impairment, length of hospital stay, duration and complexity of rehabilitative therapies, and the time after injury until visual testing.

Despite the variability in injury and recovery time, subjects displayed one or more characteristics consistent with Post-Trauma Vision Syndrome. None of the subjects had a distance prescription prior to injury. Only one

Table 1a. Visual Complaints of Patients with TBI				
Patient	Age at Testing (years)	Gender	Time Lapsed Since Injury (years)	Physical Symptoms/Vision Complaints
JU	29	M	10.5	Light sensitivity to all bright light sources Fluctuating near vision Frontal headaches with bright light or loud noises
LS	35	F	3.0	Light sensitivity to all bright light sources Blurred vision and loss of place while reading Headache with bright light or with reading
BB	42	M	2.9	Light sensitivity to outdoor light Poor dark adaptation Headache when reading
DB	41	M	1.8	Light sensitivity especially to fluorescent light Fluctuating distance and near vision Global headache with bright light
RS	35	F	0.9	Light sensitivity to outdoor light and fluorescent light Blurred vision, tearing and headache when reading
MJC	38	F	0.8	Light sensitivity to all bright light sources Tearing with > 2 min. of reading from computer monitor
APB	41	F	0.4	Light sensitivity to outdoor lighting Reading with effort > 1 min. with reading glasses

subject reported use of a near vision correction prior to examination. For best correction to 20/20 visual acuity, five subjects received a distance correction. Five subjects demonstrated a receded nearpoint of convergence, while six required a near correction for reading. Ocular health was normal (near normal for DB). All vision complaints developed soon after the TBI and persisted up to the vision examination date.

Although this was a very heterogeneous group both in terms of reported functional impairment and the duration of recovery prior to testing, none of the subjects reported any pre-morbid health or visual problems. There was no statistical difference by age between control and experimental groups. Experimental subjects reported similar educational levels compared to controls (three high school and four college graduates) and were gender-matched to controls.

Materials
Three Corning Photochromic Filters were used: CPF 450-S, 527-S and 550-S. Table 2 contains characteristics of the three CPF filters used in this study. These filters are commercially available, highly characterized and

Table 1b. Optometric Examination Data on Patients with TBI			
Patient	VA	Binocular Status	Ocular Health
JU	OD 20/20 OS 20/20	Convergence > 5 inches +1.00D add for stable reading	Anterior and posterior segments normal
LS	OD 20/20 OS 20/20	Convergence > 5 inches +1.50D add for stable reading	Anterior and posterior segments normal
BB	OD 20/20 OS 20/20	Convergence > 5 inches +1.50D add for stable reading	Anterior and posterior segments normal
DB	OD 20/20 OS 20/20	Convergence > 5 inches +1.00D add for stable reading	Small corneal scar OS 1+ NS OU
RS	OD 20/20 OS 20/20	Convergence < 5 inches +1.00D add for stable near vision	Anterior and posterior segments normal
MJC	OD 20/20 OS 20/20	Convergence < 5 inches No reading add useful, print appears "crowded" or "busy"	Anterior and posterior segments normal
APB	OD 20/20 OS 20/20	Convergence > 5 inches +1.50D add for near vision tasks	Anterior and posterior segments normal

standardized, and are of high optical quality. Since all testing was done indoors without exposure to UV light or cold temperature, the photochromic properties of these lenses were not a factor.

Procedures
Contrast sensitivity (CS)

The Pelli-Robson Letter CS Chart was selected for its ease of administration and its use of letters versus sine-wave gratings. The chart consists of 16 triplets of black letters that subtend a visual angle of $3°$ (at 1 m) and range in contrast from approximately 96 to 1%. Each successive triplet of letters differs in contrast by about 0.15 log units. Testing was performed binocularly at a viewing distance of one meter with subjects corrected for the test distance. Chart illumination was standardized at 80–90 $cd/m.^2$ The CS score was determined by the lowest triplet in which the subject correctly identified at least two letters. Scores were recorded as log contrast sensitivity.

All subjects were first tested without the filtering lenses and then with a randomized presentation of the three CPF filters. After each test condition, the CS letter chart was reversed, and different combinations of letters at the same contrast values were presented. Subjects had no prior exposure to the

Table 2. Light-Filtering Properties of Three CPF Lenses.			
	CPF 450-S	CPF 527-S	CPF 550-S
Visible light cut-off	450 nm	527 nm	550 nm
Absorption below cut-off	96%	98%	98%
Maximum transmittance above cut-off	73%	34%	26%

Data are from manufacturer (Corning Medical Optics) and from Faye, E.E. (ed.) Clinical Low Vision, 2nd ed. (Boston: Little, Brown, 1984).

three filters or prior knowledge of any potential visual benefits from their use.

Reading rate

To provide a test that was comparable to normal experience, short articles on topics of general interest were selected from one local newspaper and two national magazines (9–10 point text). Texts containing technical jargon, foreign language or unfamiliar proper names were excluded. For each filter condition, the subject read three randomly-selected paragraphs (two newsprint and one magazine print passage). The order of filter addition was randomized throughout all six test runs. Subjects were seated comfortably and wore optical corrections for near vision, if necessary. Subjects were asked to read aloud as rapidly as was comfortable and to make as few mistakes as possible. Subjects were not tested for comprehension of the passages read. Words mispronounced or omitted were subtracted from totals, and rates of reading in words/min were calculated. For experimental subjects, the CPF filter used was that one which provided the greatest improvement in CS and transmitted the most light. In five out of six cases, this was the CPF 450-S. Only JU performed best with the CPF 527-S. Since no differences in CS were found with any of the CPF lenses in control group testing, the CPF 450-S lens was selected for testing of all control subjects. The possibility of practice effects was eliminated by random introduction of the optimal filter.

Statistical analysis

Split-plot ANOVA and two-tailed Dunnett *t*-tests were used to analyze the CS and reading rate data.

Contrast sensitivity testing results

Table 3 contains results of measuring letter contrast sensitivity for the two groups in the absence of filters and while viewing through each CPF filter. Under the no filter condition, six of the seven subjects with TBI exhibited normal binocular log CS values, with BB being the sole exception; the log CS value for this subject was reduced to 1.35. (At the time of testing, BB

Table 3. Binocular Log Contrast Sensitivity Data in Normal Observers and Patients with TBI				
	No Filter	(+) 450-S	(+) 527-S	(+) 550-S
Normals (n = 7)				
Mean	1.95	1.97	1.88	1.84
(SD)	(0.12)	(0.10)	(0.08)	(0.16)
Patients (n = 7)				
JU	1.95	2.10	2.25	2.10
LS	1.95	2.25	2.25	2.10
BB	1.35	1.65	1.65	1.45[a]
DB	1.95	2.10	1.95	1.95
RS	1.95	2.25	1.95	1.95
MJC	1.95	1.95	1.80	1.65
APB	1.95	2.25	2.10	1.95
Mean	1.86	2.08	1.99	1.88
(SD)	(0.23)	(0.22)	(0.23)	(0.24)

Data for normal observers are presented as means ± SD. Data for each patient are represented to emphasize effects of individual filters on contrast sensitivity. [a]For analysis of data, an estimated point for this patient was derived by the Kirk Estimation of Missing Score equation (Kirk, R.E. Experimental Design: Procedures for the Behavioral Sciences. Belmont, CA: Brooks/Cole Publishing Company, 1968).

was still exhibiting some seizure activity and loss of vision extending two to three hours and was clearly the least recovered subject.)

Absorptive filtering of light appeared to have little effect on normal subjects. However, in six of the light-sensitive subjects with TBI, at least one filter of the three tested produced an enhancement of CS, up to a twofold increase, or 0.3 log units above that obtained without the filter. The magnitude of this enhancement may reflect a ceiling effect due to the chart's design, since the 2.25 value is assigned to the last triplet of letters at the highest contrast value on the chart. The use of light-filtering lenses may, in some cases, create enhancement beyond the twofold effect.

The log contrast sensitivity scores were analyzed using a split-plot ANOVA with one between-subjects variable (groups = two levels) and one within-subjects variable (filter conditions = four levels).

Although group was not a significant factor, there was a significant difference due to filter conditions [$F\{3,36\} = 7.72$, $P < 0.01$] and, more importantly, a significant interaction of filter conditions with groups [$F\{3,36\} = 3.33$, $P < 0.05$]. Tests of simple main effects indicated that variations in contrast sensitivity across filter conditions were statistically significant only for the group of light-sensitive patients [$F \{3,36\} = 8.25, P < 0.01$]. Finally, the significant data for this group were evaluated further using post-hoc two-tailed Dunnett t-tests to compare contrast sensitivity performance without a filter to sensitivity with each of the CPF filters. These tests indicated that, when compared to their performance without a filter, contrast sensitivity in the patient group showed significant increases with both the 450-S ($P < 0.01$) and 527-S ($P < 0.05$) filters. With consideration to performance of individuals, it is noted that maximum contrast sensitivity was measured with the 450-S for five patients and with the 527-S for one patient. The final patient had identical highest sensitivity under both the no filter condition and with the 450-S filter.

Although six of seven patients had normal contrast sensitivity results prior to addition of any of the filters tested, five patients demonstrated performance with one or more of the filters in place which was actually higher than that achieved by control subjects under identical conditions; these patients appeared to exhibit an exaggerated response to the selective effect of light absorption, especially below 450 nm. (Exaggerated cone-mediated pathway activity in TBI-induced light sensitivity is discussed later.)

Reading rate test results

During the optometric examination, each of the subjects with TBI remarked on the obvious and immediate effect that introducing the optimal filter had on his or her ability to view and read conventional text. Subjective responses included a perceived enhancement of print clarity and contrast, print that looked less "crowded," and a facilitating of eye movements thereby making reading easier. To support these subjective findings, reading rates with no filter or with the preferred filter were measured. Subjects requiring optical nearpoint correction (see Table 1b) wore the correction to read each passage. Data for the seven subjects demonstrated significant improvements with the maximal filter for each patient; because of patients' enthusiastic responses to filter use while reading, these data were expanded to include similar patients with TBI-induced light sensitivity. Results of reading performance with or without CPF 450-S filters are presented in Table 4. These data are expressed as mean $\pm$SD performance over three test passages. Data were also analyzed using the split-plot ANOVA.

Tests of simple main effects indicated that although subjects with TBI read the passages slower than normals both with a filter ($P < 0.05$) and without ($P < 0.01$), their reading rates were significantly faster ($P < 0.01$) with the filter (mean = 184.05 words/minute) as compared to reading without it (mean = 136.5 words/minute). Normals had no differences across the two conditions (210.65 with filter versus 203.91 without filter). It should be

152

Table 4. Filter Effects on Reading Rate		
	No Filter	With Filter
Normals (n = 25)		
Mean	210.65	203.91
(SD)	(13.20)	(9.25)
Patients with TBI (n = 25)		
Mean	136.5	184.05
(SD)	(25.27)	(23.34)

Data were collected as outlined in the text and are expressed as means ± standard deviations (SD) in words/minute with and without the CPF 450-S filter.

noted that everyone in the patient group improved when using the filter; relative improvements, using the no filter condition as the base, ranged from 25 to 39% with a mean of 30%.

We questioned the effects of short wavelength light absorption on reading rate. Specifically, was the enhancement in performance due to selective light absorption or to the overall reduction in light intensity? Additionally, for some patients, the inherent alteration in color perception while using this lens was aesthetically unacceptable, and the question of light reduction being provided by a non-color-distorting lens was raised. A neutral density (gray) filter that was luminance-matched to the CPF 450-S (without photochromic effect; 73% transmittance) was used to test this hypothesis. Data in Table 5 for LS and MJC suggest that overall light reduction as provided by neutral gray filters may create improvements in reading rate for some patients which equals or exceeds that seen with absorptive filtration of light with cut-off at 450 nm. Interestingly, these two subjects were the only subjects out of the original seven patients who demonstrated this effect; use of the neutral density filter during reading rate testing of the other five patients provided no effect on their reading performance.

Prescription and dispensing of these CPF lenses for all indoor tasks, for driving and for some outdoor activities has met with excellent compliance. Each subject reported wearing the lenses up to a year past dispensing. Effects initially observed have persisted, including control of light sensitivity, reduced or alleviated headache, epiphora and fatigue, and facilitated reading. Symptoms reappear when filters are not used. Since testing conditions simulated only indoor lighting and activities, additional filtering in the form of a neutral gray clip-on lens has been used successfully in bright outdoor illumination by subjects who preferred the CPF 450-S for indoor tasks.

Table 5. Filter Effects on Reading Rate for Two Patients			
Patients	No Filter	CPF 450-S	ND Filter
LS	120.5	168.3	157.8
MJC	130.2	135.1	179.3

Data were collected as outlined in the text and are expressed in words/minutes, in the absence or presence of the CPF 450-S or luminance-matched ND filter for the two individuals whose initial reading rates (no filter) improved with the ND filters.

Pupillary responses in patients with TBI

The previous discussion of some patients' preference and improved reading performance with neutral (gray) density filters provokes a comment about pupillary responses to light after TBI. Patients represented here had clinically normal pupillary reflexes as reported by their referring neurologists/ophthalmologists and as documented during slit lamp examinations. However, the parasympathetic component of the third cranial nerve controlling pupillary responses can be easily damaged during mild traumatic brain injury; moreover, approximately 20% of the nerve fiber layer from the retina does not extend back to the chiasm and lateral geniculate nucleus, but traverses down to the midbrain and the superior colliculus to gate pupillary reflexes and coordination of eye movements.[20] These fibers are also easily damaged during head trauma. It is common to observe patients after TBI who present with newly large, often asymmetrical pupils, which may fluctuate daily or hourly. These represent significantly altered tonic or resting pupillary diameters, which correlate with the aberrant, often fluctuating convergence and accommodative tone also demonstrated. Patients with these atypical pupillary characteristics complain of sensitivity to all types of intense lighting, regardless of wavelength composition. Not surprisingly, these patients respond best to overall light reduction as provided by neutral gray filters; short wavelength light filtration often appears to be too "bright" or "glaring" and is poorly tolerated.

Wavelength-specific therapy

Our data with CPF lenses suggest that at least for light-sensitive patients with normal pupillary responses, the filter of choice is the yellow CPF 450-S; approximations of these filters have been used successfully by tinting plastic lenses to approximate this wavelength specificity or by using clip-on or wraparound filters whose color components are only generally in the range of the CPF 450-S spectral composition (i.e., the yellow family). Since the mid-1980s however, much has been written regarding wavelength-specific therapeutic lenses and the highly individualized chromaticity parameters that may be necessary for maximal effects. Irlen[21] reported that some people experience perceptual distortions (e.g., movement of letters, changes in spacing and blurring of text) along with symptoms of discomfort when reading; these symptoms abated when the text had a particular color. Wilkins et al.[22] have reported a double-masked, placebo-controlled trial of precision spectral filters in children who experienced eye strain and headache while reading and who used colored overlays to advantage. The experimental design of this study addressed whether benefits of tinted lenses were attributable to placebo effects alone and whether maximally-effective tints needed to be determined with precision. Children included in this study had previously used colored theater acetate overlays for reduction in reading difficulty and asthenopia; interestingly, many children had migraine present in the family. Significant reductions in symptoms were found only when a highly idiosyncratic therapeutic tint was used, thus suggesting a real effect.

The physiologic basis of the efficacy of spectrally-precise tints is unknown. Tints have been used to reduce epileptic photosensitivity.[23] In some patients, the trigger involves focal cortical hyperexcitability;[24] minimal cortical hyperexcitability has been proposed as a neurologic basis for visual discomfort and perceptual distortions in people without epilepsy,[25] particularly those with migraine.[26] These observations are consistent with the idea that tinted lenses may reduce sensitivity to light-induced excitation of hyperexcitable regions along the visual pathways. This hypothesis might be generalized to include other categories of patients with light-induced visual symptoms, including patients with TBI. The loci of injury responsible for this proposed increased photic-driven hyperexcitability in patients with TBI is obscure, but would appear to be, at the very least, postretinal. Freed and Hellerstein[27] have reported on the normal electroretinographic (ERG) responses of patients with mild TBI who, nonetheless, demonstrated significantly abnormal pattern visual evoked potential (VEP) amplitudes. Padula et al.[11] have confirmed the presence of anomalous VEP responses in patients with mild TBI, which are remediable by vision therapies including binasal occlusion and small amounts of base-in prism.

It is unknown whether tinted lenses can also modify and/or normalize VEPs in patients with TBI who have visual symptoms of PTVS including light sensitivity. However, Riddell et al[28] have reported a preliminary study assessing the effects of colored lenses on the VEP responses measured in children with light sensitivity of heterogeneous etiology. With regard to differences in VEP responses to colored lenses, the presence or absence of migraine headache correlated significantly with the VEP outcome; children with migraine showed far more objective differences in VEP measures with or without colored lenses than those children without migraine who experienced similar visual symptoms abated by use of tinted lenses. The small sample size of this intriguing study excludes any generalizations about wavelength-specific alterations in postretinal responses to light. However, some patients with TBI experience subsequent migraine-type symptoms including disabling light sensitivity, phonophobia, etc. Further examination of response similarities between groups of migraineurs and patients with mild TBI may reveal common mechanisms of action and loci of injury responsible for visual symptoms, leading to the development of novel treatment regimens, including wavelength-specific therapies.

Dark adaptation

During the course of our investigation and treatment of light sensitivity with light-filtering lenses, some patients reported the continued successful use of filters in lighted environments, but completely rejected their use in dim illumination. Even after removing these filters, they noted significant losses in visual functioning in the dark. Although approximately 90% of examined TBI patients spontaneously reported an acute onset of significant light sensitivity, coincident reports of anomalous dark adaptability were far less frequent, even after direct inquiry. To quantify the apparently paradoxical complaint of poor dark adaptation and detect its true frequency in this population, standardized clinical dark adaptometry was performed on patients with TBI-induced light sensitivity at different stages of recovery. Three groups of patients were examined; categories of patients were based on the degree of light sensitivity at the time of testing. These included patients with A) profound, persistent light sensitivity one to three years past injury, B) moderate light sensitivity which, although intense at onset, had decreased during the first six months to two years past injury, and C) mild or absent light sensitivity, which was significantly acute after injury, but resolved rapidly within the first weeks/months after injury (0.3-0.5 months).

Methods
Subjects

Fifty control subjects, 20 males and 30 females ranging from 14–50 years of age, were recruited from staff at SUNY Health Science Center. Ten patients with documented TBI, four males and six females, 22-45 years of age, 0.3 to 3.0 years past injury, were selected from patients referred for optometric evaluation. All subjects were given complete vision examinations; all subjects had normal ocular health including clinically normal pupillary responses, were receiving no medications known to alter visual responses, including light sensitivity, were corrected to 20/20 in each eye, and demonstrated no defects in visual fields of either eye with confrontational field testing. No attempt was made to grade the actual level of traumatic brain injury either at the time of trauma or at the time of vision testing. Some patients were still receiving outpatient therapies and/or had returned to work. All patients were ambulatory, articulated well, and demonstrated understanding of test procedures prior to test runs, which were constantly monitored. Table 6 contains various characteristics and vision complaints of TBI patients included in this study.

Dark Adaptometry (DA)

All subjects were optically corrected for the test distance and were tested monocularly (OD), with the nontested eye patched. Some patients were also tested binocularly (i.e., BB, JS, LC-G, KA). Pupils remained undilated. Subjects were placed in a Goldmann-Weekers dark adaptometer ganzfeld. After two minutes of pre-adaptation with eyes closed, each subject viewed the illuminated bowl at 1400 cd/m^2 for five minutes. The adapting field was then turned off and threshold measurements were recorded for the next 30 minutes according to the standard Goldmann-Weekers procedure. A centrally-presented, circular, flashing, 10°, 500 msec, white test stimulus was presented once per second. Measurements were made approximately three times/minute, using the ascending method-of-limits. Figure 1 contains the response curve for data obtained from 50 normal subjects.

Figures 2a-4a contain dark adaptation curves of three representative patients in group A who expressed profound, disabling light sensitivity after injury, which had persisted up to the time of testing (1.0 to 3.0 years past injury). Each of these patients benefited from light-filtering lenses both indoors and outdoors and used them routinely. Each patient also remarked on their significant problem with visual tasks under low levels of illumination, which appear to be coincident with the onset of post-traumatic light sensitivity. JR and JP reported making the decision to curtail or eliminate driving at night, despite the absence of any such recommendations from their treating clinicians. JS also noted poor night vision; supplementary lighting at night had become essential for safety, even at home. Results of dark adaptometry for this group were striking. Maximal cone-mediated thresholds were elevated 0.4 to 1.3 log units as compared to control responses, while rod-mediated sensitivity was reduced to an even greater extent, with maximal thresholds elevated 1.3 to 2.3 log units above control values. Results of repeated testing of JR, 3 months later, are included in Figure 2a for comparison; they confirm the initial observations of >2 log unit losses in rod sensitivity.

	Patient	Gender	Age at Testing (years)	Time Since Injury (years)	Vision Complaints
					Table 6. Characteristics of patients with TBI.
A	JR	M	44	1.0	Profound light sensitivity; poor night driving; day driving appears "tunnel-like"
	JP	M	45	3.0	Moderate-profound light sensitivity; night driving very difficult
	BB	M	43	1.0	Profound light sensitivity; "gets lost in the dark;" prolonged dark adaptation
	JS	F	28	2.3	Profound light sensitivity; reduced peripheral field awareness; vision "poor" in dim illumination
B	JH	F	26	0.5	Moderate light sensitivity; visual "clutter" is distracting, especially while driving; no dark-adaptive problems noted
	VK	F	31	1.8	Fluctuating moderate light sensitivity; problems driving in city traffic
	LC-G	F	22	1.6	Moderate-mild light sensitivity; night vision "O.K.;" has returned to some daylight driving
C	RS	M	25	0.3	Acute-profound light sensitivity after injury now resolved; no night vision problems; driving comfortable
	KA	F	31	0.5	Mild light sensitivity to sunlight; no night vision problems; has returned to driving
	WA	F	26	0.4	Moderate light sensitivity noticed initially now almost resolved; dark adaptation appears normal; not yet driving

Categories of patients are based on the level of light sensitivity reported: A) profound light sensitivity (JR, JP, BB, JS), B) moderate light sensitivity (JH, VK, LC-G) and C) mild/absent light sensitivity (RS, KA, WA).

Figure 5a contains results of dark adaptometry for one representative patient in group B, 0.5 years past injury, who at the time of testing complained of moderate light sensitivity; patients in group B used light-filtering lenses only situationally. However, a review of clinical histories documented that each of these patients had experienced an intense light sensitivity immediately after injury, with appreciable reduction in light sensitivity during the subsequent six to twelve months past TBI. Additionally, although these patients did not note visual losses in the dark, two of the three complained of reduced peripheral vision, especially while driving. Maximal cone- and rod-mediated threshold differences from control values for this group were less dramatic than those exhibited by patients in group A; cone-mediated responses were elevated 0.3 to 0.4 log units above

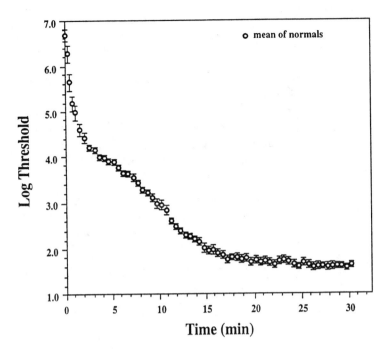

Figure 1. Dark adaptation response curve for 50 control subjects. 20 male and 30 female subjects, 14-50 years of age, were recruited from staff at State University of New York Health Science Center (SUNY HSC). Subjects were tested as outlined in Methods. Symbols indicate mean values ± standard deviation (SD) values. Threshold luminance (in log units) is plotted throughout a testing period of 30 minutes. The overall range of sensitivity achieved by these subjects was approximately 5 log units; the initial rapid recovery of sensitivity (cone-mediated) accounted for approximately 2.5 log units. After 5 minutes of recovery, rod-mediated responses became active and allowed for an additional 2.5 log units of sensitivity recovery.

control values, whereas rod-mediated responses demonstrated a two to threefold greater reduction in sensitivity, with maximal threshold differences from controls ranging from 0.7 to 1.1 log units.

Figure 6a demonstrates dark adaptometry tracings for one patient in group C who, at the time of testing, had recovered from much of the visual consequences of his brain injury. Patients in Group C all admitted to an acute onset of intense light sensitivity after injury as well as some peripheral visual field reductions, much of which had rapidly resolved in 0.3 to 0.5 months. These patients noted little atypical light sensitivity at the time of testing; dark adaptation or peripheral vision reductions were not reported. Maximal cone- and rod-mediated thresholds were elevated only 0.1 to 0.2 log units and 0.2 to 0.5 log units, respectively.

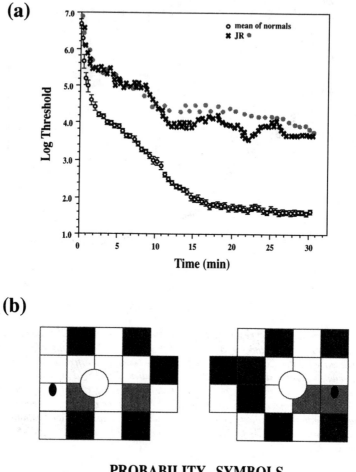

(a)

(b)

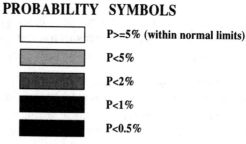

PROBABILITY SYMBOLS

P>=5% (within normal limits)

P<5%

P<2%

P<1%

P<0.5%

Figure 2a and b. JR, a 44-year-old white male, 1.0 years past injury; TBI with subsequent significant light sensitivity; neuroimaging documented cervical strain. Dark adaptometry and threshold visual field analysis conducted as outlined in Methods. a) Maximal threshold differences from control values: −1.2 log units (cone); -2.30 log units (rod). b) Visual field indices: mean deviation (OD) −0.72 and (OS) −0.70 log units; fixation errors 0/6 OU; false negatives 0/5 OU; false positives 0/8 OU.

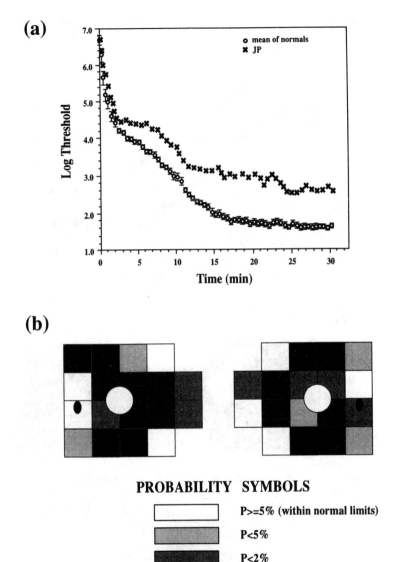

(a)

(b)

PROBABILITY SYMBOLS

P>=5% (within normal limits)

P<5%

P<2%

P<1%

P<0.5%

Figure 3a and b. JP, a 45-year-old white male, 3.0 years past injury; TBI with subsequent profound light sensitivity; normal neuroimaging results. Dark adaptometry and threshold visual field analysis conducted as outlined in Methods. a) Maximal threshold differences from control values: –0.5 log units (cone); –1.2 log units (rod). b) Visual field indices: mean deviation (OD) –0.95 and (OS) –0.89 log units; fixation errors 0/6 OU; false negatives 0/5 OU; false positives 0/8 OU.

(a)

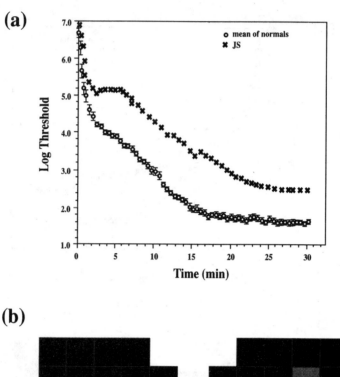

(b)

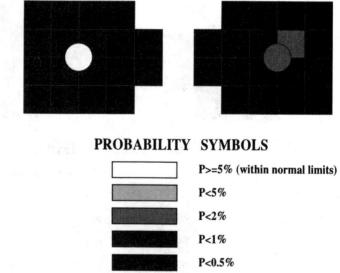

Figure 4a and b. *JS, a 28-year-old white female, 2.3 years past injury; TBI with profound light sensitivity; normal neuroimaging results. Dark adaptometry and threshold visual field analysis conducted as outlined in Methods. a) Maximal threshold differences from control values: −1.1 log units (cone); −1.8 log units (rod). b) Visual field indices: mean deviation (OD) −1.70 and OS −1.57 log units; fixation errors 0/6 OU; false negatives 0/5 OU; false positives 0/8 OU.*

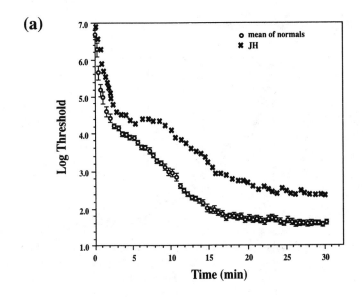

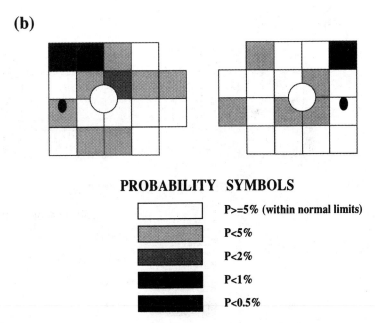

Figure 5a and b. JH, a 26-year-old white female, 0.5 years past injury; TBI with moderate light sensitivity; normal neuroimaging results. Dark adaptometry and threshold visual field analysis conducted as outlined in Methods. a) Maximal threshold differences from control values: –0.40 log units (cone); –1.17 log units (rod). b) Visual field indices: mean deviation (OD) –0.29 and (OS) –0.44 log units; fixation errors 0/6 OD, 1/6 OS; false negatives 0/5 OU; false positives 0/8 OU.

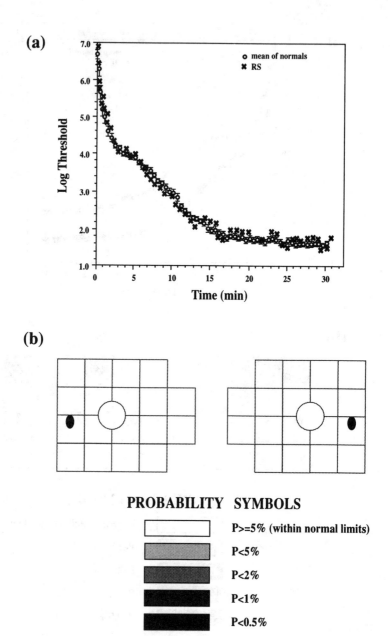

(a)

(b)

PROBABILITY SYMBOLS

P>=5% (within normal limits)

P<5%

P<2%

P<1%

P<0.5%

Figure 6a and b. RS, a 25-year-old white male, 0.3 years past injury; TBI with subsequent rapid resolution of light sensitivity; normal neuroimaging results. Dark adaptometry and visual field analysis conducted as outlined in Methods. a) Maximal threshold differences from control values: −0.1 log units (cone); −0.2 log units (rod). b) Visual field indices: mean deviation (OD) +0.24 and (OS) +0.25 log units; fixation errors 0/6 OU; false negatives 0/5 OU; false positives 0/8 OU.

Table 7. Dark Adaptation in Patients with TBI.		
	Maximal Threshold Differences From Control Values	
Group	Cone Threshold (log units)	Rod Threshold (log units)
A	-0.80 ± 0.41	-1.63 ± 0.53
B	-0.37 ± 0.06	-0.90 ± 0.20
C	-0.13 ± 0.06	-0.37 ± 0.15

Data are from three groups of patients with A profound, B moderate, or C mild/absent light sensitivity expressed at the time of testing. Maximal threshold differences were estimated from recorded tracings and are expressed in log units. Negative values indicate reduction in sensitivity as compared to controls. Data are expressed as means ± SD.

Table 7 contains a summary of cone- and rod-mediated responses for the three groups of patients who underwent dark adaptometry. A two to three-fold greater loss in rod-mediated activity as compared to cone response levels was a surprisingly consistent finding throughout the three groups of patients.

Given the magnitude of rod-mediated sensitivity losses found in each group of patients and the common complaint of losses in peripheral visual field awareness, we elected to expand testing beyond the central $10°$ field assessed by dark adaptometry to include visual sensitivity throughout the central $30°$ fields.

Visual Field Testing

A Humphrey Systems Frequency Doubling Technology full threshold test (N-30 stimulus presentation pattern) was performed monocularly, with the patient's habitual visual correction in place and pupils undilated. Corrective lenses were untinted, and the nontested eye was not patched but was unaligned with the viewed testing window. The 19 location stimulus presentation pattern consisted of four $10°$ square targets per quadrant and a central $5°$ radius target; two additional $10°$ targets were presented above and below the horizontal midline between $20°$ and $30°$ in each nasal visual field. Stimuli consisted of flickering black and white vertical bars of low spatial frequency (0.25 cycles/degree) and high temporal frequency (25 Hz counterphase flicker) designed to stimulate retinal ganglion cells in the magnocellular (M-cell) pathway. Background luminance level was 60-70 cd/m.^{2} The location of targets is illustrated in Figure 7.

Each patient observed a brief demonstration of the testing procedure prior to the actual test run. Stimuli were presented randomly at 19 different retinal locations. Simultaneous staircases were determined for each location by the system computer. False positive errors were checked by randomly presenting a blank trial (zero contrast). False negative errors were checked by presenting a stimulus at maximal contrast (100%). Fixation losses were

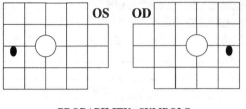

OS OD

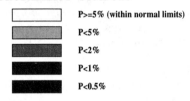

PROBABILITY SYMBOLS

P>=5% (within normal limits)

P<5%

P<2%

P<1%

P<0.5%

Figure 7. The 19 location stimulus presentation pattern of the Humphrey Systems Frequency Doubling Technology Full Threshold (N-30) Test.

monitored by periodically presenting a small target in the blind spot. Data were analyzed using the statistical package available with the instrument, which uses an age and eye-adjusted normative database to calculate various visual field indices. Mean deviation (MD) was one index provided which represented the average sensitivity of all 19 stimulus locations in comparison to the average, normative response, providing an indication of overall field sensitivity. Patterns of losses were represented by a gray scale indicating whether the sensitivity for an individual test point was normal or whether it fell below the lower 5%, 2%, 1%, or 0.5% of the normal, age-related population.

Figures 2b-4b contain gray scale representations of results of visual field perimetry for the three patients in group A previously cited. Each patient demonstrated significant visual field sensitivity losses throughout the central 30 degrees, with each patient exhibiting a constriction of the field for each eye with preservation of sensitivity in the central ten degrees. During testing, each patient remarked that they had experienced a momentary "collapsing" or "darkening" of the test field, despite preservation of central field vision (i.e., the fixation dot was always in view). This reduction in field brightness began at the edges of the field and increased with time, often encompassing most of the test field area. Brief rests or eye closures restored field brightness.

Figure 5b shows results of visual field testing for JH, the patient representing group B responses. The gray scale representation shows scattered moderate/mild losses in sensitivity throughout the central 30 degrees. Each group B patient also reported brief episodes of field obscuration and dimming of field brightness, which became progressively more apparent with time and were alleviated with eye closures.

Figure 6b contains results of visual field testing for RS in group C. Two of the three patients, RS and KA, had completely normal visual field results.

WA's visual field testing revealed only mild/moderate scattered losses in the right eye; the left visual field was completely normal.

Table 8 contains averages of the entire visual field of each right eye, expressed as mean deviation in log units, to facilitate a direct comparison to log unit changes in rod thresholds for right eyes of the same patient. (Very little variation was seen in visual field sensitivity between the two eyes). A linear regression analysis of data based on right eye mean deviation field sensitivity versus rod thresholds for each patient is plotted in Figure 8. This figure clearly shows the strong relationship between peripheral visual field sensitivity and rod-mediated sensitivity.

Conclusions
Mechanisms of altered visual adaptation
Sensory adaptation to the wide range of luminance levels encountered in daily living is critical for normal visual functioning, because it allows visual sensitivity to remain stable, regardless of the level of ambient illumination. Traditionally, visual adaptation has been attributed to retinal processes.[29-30] However, reports by patients with posterior brain damage have included visual responses to natural levels of light which are often characterized as "blinding" or "dim/dark" and, for each case, disabling.[31] Results of our previous studies and of those reported here demonstrate that:

1. patients who have sustained TBI often experience a new, intense, chronic light sensitivity, which may resolve spontaneously within the first weeks/months past injury or which may persist for years;

2. this light sensitivity may be present despite normal ocular health, pupillary function, non-interference from systemic disease or medication, negative results of neuroimaging and normal confrontational visual field testing;

3. light sensitivity in patients with TBI can be successfully treated with one or more light-filtering lenses; use of these filters can improve visual performance (enhance contrast sensitivity and reading rate) and reduce or eliminate the consequences of an exaggerated response of the cone-mediated pathway (photic-driven headache, visual/perceptual distortions, asthenopia, etc.);

4. all of the patients we have currently tested who complained of light sensitivity also demonstrated significant losses in dark adaptation and visual field sensitivity; results of DA testing documented two to threefold greater reductions in rod-mediated sensitivity as compared to cone-mediated responses;

Table 8.

Results of Dark Adaptometry (DA) and Visual Field Testing of Patients with TBI.

	Patient	Maximal Rod Threshold Differences from Controls (log units)	Average Visual Field Differences from Controls (log units)
		(OD)	(OD)
A	JR	-2.3	-0.72
	JP	-1.2	-0.95
	BB	-1.2	-1.04
	JS	-1.8	-1.70
	mean ± s.d.	-1.63 ± 0.53	-1.10 ± 0.42
B	JH	-1.1	-0.29
	VK	-0.9	-0.28
	LC-G	-0.7	-0.47
	mean ± s.d.	-0.90 ± 0.20	-0.35 ± 0.11
C	RS	-0.2	+0.24
	KA	-0.5	+0.24
	WA	-0.4	-0.27
	mean ± s.d.	-0.37 ± 0.15	+0.07 ± 0.29

For DA, maximal threshold response differences from controls were estimated from re-corded tracings. Average visual field sensitivity difference from controls is the mean deviation (MD) or average sensitivity of all 19 stimulus locations as compared to age-adjusted normals, calculated by the statistical package accompanying the perimeter. Positive/negative values indicate sensitivity that is better/worse than the control or average, normal observer. Categories of patients based on levels of light sensitivity reported: A) profound, B) moderate, C) mild/absent.

5. patients who reported no light sensitivity at the time of testing demonstrated DA responses and visual field results that were at or near normal levels. These data suggest that the presence of light sensitivity after TBI may be predictive of coincident problems with peripheral field sensitivity.

Three broad categories of patients have emerged from these studies: A) patients who have persistent (>1 year past injury), profound light sensitivity with marked losses in dark adaptation and field sensitivity, and who note considerable functional problems with visual tasks in dim illumination or those requiring peripheral field awareness (mobility, driving, etc); B) patients with moderate, situational light sensitivity sustained six months or longer, whose reductions on DA and visual field testing are approximately half that of patients in group A, and who noted more limited complaints about peripheral awareness without identifying particular problems with dark environments and; C) patients who have experienced a rapid visual re-

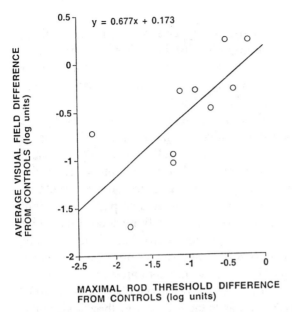

$$y = 0.677x + 0.173$$

AVERAGE VISUAL FIELD DIFFERENCE FROM CONTROLS (log units)

MAXIMAL ROD THRESHOLD DIFFERENCE FROM CONTROLS (log units)

Figure 8. Graphical presentation of the linear regression analysis of data comparing right eye mean deviation field sensitivity and rod threshold values for the ten patients included in the study.

covery from TBI, with mild/absent light sensitivity remaining after four to six months, with little or no effect on dark adaptation or visual field sensitivity.

Despite differences in patient populations and methodology, our results can be compared to those of Zihl and Kerkhoff,[14] who reported impaired foveal photopic and scotopic adaptation in a large number of patients with unilateral or bilateral postgeniculate brain damage of various etiologies. As with our results, all patients in that study who complained of visual adaptation disturbances demonstrated quantifiable impaired adaptive responses upon testing; normal subjects or brain-damaged patients who lacked complaints tested normally. Furthermore, patients who demonstrated reduced scotopic adaptation often did not report impaired vision in dim illumination or periods of "dark" vision. In our study, patients in group B, all of whom reported moderate light sensitivity, did not identify problems with low levels of light, despite the fact that each showed significant losses in cone- and rod-mediated responses as compared to controls during DA testing. In addition, each patient in group A spontaneously reported profound light sensitivity as a striking visual disability, but three of the four patients admitted to reduced visual capacity in the dark only after detailed interrogation, despite the often dramatic quantitative losses in sensitivity seen during DA testing. Clinicians should be aware of the greater tendency to report abnormal photopic versus scotopic sensitivity and be ready to address this disparity with detailed history taking directed toward issues of ambient lighting and visual functioning.

Reduction in rod-mediated sensitivity seen in group A correlated well with patient complaints of visual dysfunction in the dark. However, patients complaining of light sensitivity also demonstrated losses in cone-mediated activity. What, then, is the mechanism for hypersensitivity to light in these patients? Data in Table 7 demonstrated that in each group of patients tested, rod-mediated activity had been reduced two to threefold greater than cone-mediated activity. Since cone- and rod-mediated pathways are thought to be mutually antagonistic,[32] the far greater reduction in rod-mediated responses may allow for an exaggerated response by the cone pathway to suprathreshold stimulation by light. This same disinhibition of central, cone-mediated (parvocellular) activity may help explain our previous findings of supranormal or hyper contrast sensitivity in patients with TBI who utilized light-filtering lenses. Another explanation for the hyperresponsiveness of the cone-mediated pathway to light stimulation, despite reductions in cone-mediated activity documented with dark adaptometry, may be found in the phenomenon of recruitment in auditory dysfunction.[33] Recruitment is defined as an abnormal growth or incremental change in loudness for signals at suprathreshold intensities perceived by impaired ears. Normally, auditory nerve fibers responsive to characteristic frequencies (CF) vary as to their respective threshold; as the intensity of a given frequency is increased, more and more fibers with that CF respond. In the impaired ear, nerve fibers are thought to be more broadly tuned; as signal intensity is increased at a given CF, fibers with higher CFs will also respond more than would be expected under normal conditions. Recruitment is therefore a response to damage which broadens or increases the sensitivity of remaining nerve fibers to the same signal intensity. With regard to TBI-induced losses in cone-mediated activity, a similar recruitment of undamaged cone (parvocellular) fibers may take place at suprathreshold light levels, producing a perceived hyperstimulation and photophobia.

Visual adaptation and the brain

An understanding of the mechanisms underlying light sensitivity and reduced dark adaptation would be facilitated by identifying the loci of injury in these patients. With regard to DA testing, no attempt was made to control pupillary responses or restrict diameters, and although pupillary function in all patients was clinically normal, direct observation of pupillary function during testing was not made. However, even if abnormal pupillary responses were associated with impaired adaptation, this would support an hypothesis of a contribution of a postretinal mechanism to visual adaptation.

Our preliminary results of fluorescein angiography performed on patients with TBI who were profoundly light sensitive do not support a role for retinal ischemia as a mechanism producing trauma-induced light sensitivity. With traumatic brain injury, there may be a massive release of catecholamines from the adrenal glands, creating vascular constriction. Imaging of the retinal vascular network throughout all phases of arteriovenous filling demonstrated completely normal perfusion rates; no areas of dye leakage or abnormal retinal perfusion were observed. However, studies with single-photon emission computer tomography (SPECT)[34] have demonstrated brain hypoperfusion in greater than half of tested patients who demonstrated chronic postconcussion symptoms, such as headache and memory loss; similar findings have been noted in patients after mild trauma or whiplash.[35-36] In each case, results of conventional magnetic resonance imaging (MRI) or computer tomography (CT) scan were normal. Results of neuroimaging in our patients were not predictive of visual deficit: three out of four patients in group A with profound visual adaptation impairment had normal MRI and CT scans. In the future, high resolution functional imaging may provide answers concerning locations of injury and mechanisms of visual impairment. Currently, more compelling evidence is the visual electrodiagnostic reports of Freed and Hellerstein[27] who used full-field electroretinography (ERG) and visually-evoked cortical potentials (VECP) to assess patients with mild TBI. ERG results were unremarkable and insensitive for detection of TBI. VECP results, however, did allow for identification of visual pathway dysfunction; a large majority of TBI patients in that study showed waveform abnormalities. Similar reports were cited by Padula et al.[11] who reported significant reductions in (N1-P1) amplitudes of visual evoked potentials in patients after brain trauma. It is important to note that two patients in group A (BB, JS) and one patient each in groups B (LC-G) and C (KA) were tested under both monocular and binocular viewing conditions for DA testing; results were essentially identical for each viewing condition, supporting the possible involvement of visual pathway activity beyond the retina in creating impaired responses. Additionally, the high degree of correlation found between visual field sensitivity losses and losses found in rod-mediated activity upon DA testing is suggestive of common postretinal mechanisms and/or loci of injury mediating these effects.

To date, the best single predictor of quantifiable reductions in visual adaptation in brain-injured patients is found in patient reports received during careful history taking. This observation emphasizes the necessity of clinicians listening to patients' complaints and asking questions concerning their responses to illumination levels encountered during daily living activities.

References

1. Sosin DM, Sniezek JE, Thurman, DJ. Incidence of mild and moderate brain injury in the United States, 1991. Brain Injury 1996;10(1):47-54.

171

2. Kraus J, Sorenson S. Epidemiology. In: Silver J, Yadofsky S, Hales R, eds. Neuropsychiatry of Traumatic Brain Injury. Washington, DC: American Psychiatric Press, Inc., 1994.

3. Sosin DM, Sniezek JE, Waxweiler RJ. Trends in death associated with traumatic brain injury, 1979 through 1992: success and failure. J Am Med Assoc 1995; 273(22):1778-80.

4. Max W, MacKenzie EJ, Rice DP. Head injuries: costs and consequences. J Head Trauma Rehab 1991; 6(2):76-91.

5. Padula WV. Neuro-optometric rehabilitation for persons with TBI or CVA. J Opt Vis Dev 1992; 23:4-8.

6. Harrison RJ. Loss of fusional vergence with partial loss of accommodative convergence and accommodation following head injury. Binoc Vis 1987;2:93-100.

7. Aksionoff EB, Falk NS. The differential diagnosis of perceptual deficits in traumatic brain injury patients. J Am Optom Assoc 1992;63:554-58.

8. Tierney DW. Visual dysfunction in closed head injury. J Am Optom Assoc 1988;59:614-22

9. Hellerstein LF, Freed S, Maples WC. Vision profile of patients with mild brain injury. J Am Optom Assoc 1995;66:634-39.

10. Baker RS, Epstein AV. Ocular motor abnormalities from head trauma. Surv Ophthalmol 1991;35:245-67.

11. Padula WV, Argyris S, Ray S. Visual evoked potentials (VEP) evaluating treatment for post-trauma vision syndrome (PTVS) in patients with traumatic brain injuries (TBI). Brain Injury 1994;8:125-33.

12. Gianutsos R, Ramsey G, Perlin R. Rehabilitative optometric services for survivors of acquired brain injury. J Am Optom Assoc 1998;69:573-8.

13. Jackowski MM, Sturr JF, Taub HA, Turk MA. Photophobia in patients with traumatic brain injury: uses of light-filtering lenses to enhance contrast sensitivity and reading rate. NeuroRehab 1996;6:193-201.

14. Zihl J, Kerkhoff G. Foveal photopic and scotopic adaptation in patients with brain damage. Clini Vis Sci 1990;5(2):185-95.

15. Jackowski MM, Sturr JF, Turk MA, Friedman DI. Clinical indications of altered peripheral field function in patients with traumatic brain injury. Invest Ophthalmol Vis Sci 1999;40(4):32 (supplement).

16. Gronwall DM. Minor head injury. Neuropsych 1991;5:253-65.

17. Lebensohn JE. The nature of photophobia. Arch Ophthalmol 1934;12:380-390.

18. Waddell PA, Gronwall DM. Sensitivity to light and sound following minor head injury. Acta Neurologica Scandinavica 1984;69:270-6.

19. Bohnen S, Twijnstra A, Wijnen G et al. Tolerance for light and sound of patients with persistent post-concussional symptoms 6 months after mild head injury. Neurology 1991;238:443-6.

20. Padula WV. Vision: the process. In: Padula WV, ed. Neuro-Optometric Rehabilitation. Santa Ana, CA: Optometric Extension Program Foundation, Inc. 1996: 4-6.

21. Irlen H. Reading by the Colors. New York: Avery Press, 1991.

22. Wilkins AJ, Evans BJW, Brown JA et al. Double-masked placebo-controlled trial of precision spectral filters in children who use coloured overlays. Ophthal Physiol Opt 1994;14:365-70.

23. Newmark ME, Penry JK. Photosensitivity and Epilepsy: A Review. New York: Raven Press, 1979:128.

24. Wilkins AJ, Binnie CD, Darby CE. Visually-induced seizures. Prog Neurobiol 1980;15:85-117.

25. Wilkins AJ, Nimmo-Smith MI, Trait A et al. A neurological basis for visual discomfort. Brain 1984;107:989-1017.

26. Marcus DA, Soso MJ. Migraine and stripe-induced discomfort. Arch Neurol 1989;46:1129-32.

27. Freed S, Hellerstein LF. Visual electrodiagnostic findings in mild traumatic brain injury. Brain Injury 1997;11(1):25-36.

28. Riddell PM, Wilkins AJ, Zemon V et al. The effect of coloured lenses on the visual evoked response in photophobic children. Invest Ophthalmol Vis Sci 1998;39:181 (supplement).

29. Dowling JE. The site of visual adaptation. Sci 1967;155:273-9.

30. Shapley R, Enroth-Cugell C. Visual adaptation and retinal gain control. Progress in Retinal Res 1984;3:263-346.

31. Korner F, Teuber HL. Visual field defects after missile injuries to the geniculo-striate pathway in man. Experi Brain Res 1973;18:88-113.

32. Cohen AI. The retina. In: Hart WM, ed. Adler's Physiology of the Eye. St. Louis: Mosby Yearbook, 1992:579-615.

33. Brunt MA. Bekesy audiometry and loudness balance testing. In: Katz J, ed. Handbook of Clinical Audiology. 3rd ed. Baltimore, MD: Williams and Wilkins, 1985:281-9.

34. Bavetta S, Nimmon CC, White J et al. A prospective study comparing SPECT with MRI and CT as prognostic indicators following severe closed head injury. Nuclear Med Communications 1994;15:961-8.

35. Jacobs A, Put E, Ingels M et al. Prospective evaluation of Technetium 99m-HMPAO SPECT in mild and moderate traumatic brain injury. J Nuclear Med 1994;35:942-7.

36. Otte A, Mueller-Brand J, Fierz L. Brain SPECT findings in late whiplash syndrome. Lancet 1995;345:1513-4.

The Integration of Visual and Vestibular Systems in Balance Disorders—A Clinical Perspective

Steven A. Rosen, M.D.
Allen H. Cohen, O.D.
Stacy Trebing, P.T.

Introduction

Dizziness, vertigo and gait disturbance, and their effect on balance, are among the most common complaints for which patients seek medical attention. In the past, standard physical and rehabilitation therapy focused on the musculoskeletal system; neurologists confined their attention to disorders of the central (CNS) or peripheral nervous system, and otologists confined their attention to the peripheral vestibular system or inner ear. Recent advances in the understanding of central and peripheral vestibular function have resulted in the emergence of a rational, dynamic and comprehensive management strategy, namely vestibular rehabilitation. Similar advances have been seen in the application of central and peripheral visual physiology to balance disorders. As a result, the rehabilitation optometrist has added an important component to the overall understanding and treatment of this patient population. With this shift in focus, it has become apparent that many patients require the comprehensive integration of visual and vestibular therapies to restore balance function fully. Today, the "balance specialist" must consider the multitude of etiologies that cause balance disturbances to provide a comprehensive and rational treatment plan that has the highest likelihood of success. This chapter will discuss, in a clinically relevant format, the underlying pathophysiology, clinical features, diagnostic testing, and resulting treatment protocols based on this conceptual framework.

The Neurophysiology of Balance

To appreciate fully how these complex systems integrate to create an efficient balance system and understand how different disease processes can disrupt this system, a basic understanding of the anatomy and physiology of the balance system is important. This section summarizes the basic knowledge of vestibular neurophysiology and the established visual models, so that a comprehensive multidisciplinary approach can emerge.

At the most basic level, the balance system can be analyzed using the cybernetic concept of an input/output model. In living systems, this is referred to as the afferent-efferent model.[1] In essence, sensory afferent information (input) results in motor responses (output). The human balance system has three afferent systems: vestibular, visual and somatosensory. The efferent system consists of multiple neurological pathways that to some degree overlap and are redundant. All of these pathways ultimately affect motor responses of the limbs, trunk and eyes to maintain balance during varying environmental situations.

Because the vestibular system is the primary factor in balance, the following discussions are more fully devoted to this system than to the visual and somatosensory systems.

The vestibular system

The vestibular system (the inner ear) is usually viewed as a peripheral system that forwards information to the central vestibular system located within the CNS. The vestibular apparatus is located bilaterally within the petrous portion of the temporal bone and is part of the vestibulocochlear complex.

Subdivisions of the vestibular apparatus

The bony labyrinth is a series of hollowed cavities within the bone. Inside the bony labyrinth is the membranous labyrinth. Perilymphatic fluid separates the bony and membranous labyrinth. Endolymph is found within the membranous labyrinth.

The vestibular apparatus or labyrinth has two main subdivisions, which are sensitive to different types of head movements due to their unique anatomy. Today, our understanding of many patient symptoms as well as specific disease entities can be explained based upon this unique anatomic distinction.

The semicircular canals are ring-shaped structures that are geometrically configured to be sensitive to rotational acceleration in all directions of space (Figure 1). Thus, there are two horizontal (one in each ear) semicircular canals, two anterior semicircular canals, and two posterior semicircular canals. The dual representation of each direction of movement allows for the identification of the yaw, pitch and roll of a head movement as well as the specific direction (i.e, head turn right versus head turn left).

It is interesting to note that the exact position of the semicircular canals within the skull geometrically mirrors the functional actions of the extraocular muscles as a result of their insertion on the eyeballs. This is one reason why strabismus surgery will often need to be followed by

Vestibular Receptors

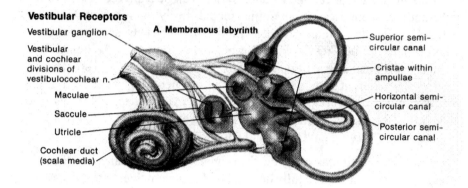

Vestibular ganglion

A. Membranous labyrinth

Vestibular and cochlear divisions of vestibulocochlear n.

Maculae

Saccule

Utricle

Cochlear duct (scala media)

Superior semi-circular canal

Cristae within ampullae

Horizontal semi-circular canal

Posterior semi-circular canal

Figure 1. Membranous labyrinth. The three semicircular canals are anatomically config-ured to detect rotational acceleration. The utricle and saccule are the otolithic structures that are sensitive to linear and gravitational acceleration. Copyright 1999, Icon Learning Systems, LLC, a subsidiary of MediMedia USA, Inc. Reprinted with permission from ICON Learning Systems, LLC, illustrated by Frank H. Netter, M.D. All rights reserved.

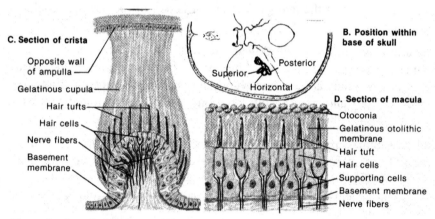

C. Section of crista

Opposite wall of ampulla

Gelatinous cupula

Hair tufts

Hair cells

Nerve fibers

Basement membrane

B. Position within base of skull

Posterior

Superior

Horizontal

D. Section of macula

Otoconia

Gelatinous otolithic membrane

Hair tuft

Hair cells

Supporting cells

Basement membrane

Nerve fibers

Figure 2. Detailed anatomy of the cristae of the semicircular canal ampullae and the macula of the otoliths. Both structures share many common features including hair cells im-bedded in a gelatinous membrane. Otoconia are unique to the otoliths which impart mass and thereby allow detection of gravitational and linear accelerating forces. Copyright 1999, Icon Learning Systems, LLC, a subsidiary of MediMedia USA, Inc. Reprinted with permis-sion from ICON Learning Systems, LLC, illustrated by Frank H. Netter, M.D. All rights re-served.

optometric vision therapy in conjunction with head and eye movement re-habilitation exercises. In effect, the CNS recalibrates the neural input from the vestibular system of the inner ears to the motor output of the extraocular muscles.

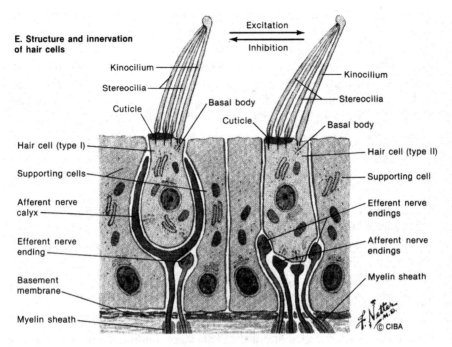

E. Structure and innervation of hair cells

Excitation

Inhibition

Kinocilium

Stereocilia

Cuticle

Basal body

Cuticle

Kinocilium

Stereocilia

Basal body

Hair cell (type I)

Supporting cells

Afferent nerve calyx

Efferent nerve ending

Basement membrane

Myelin sheath

Hair cell (type II)

Supporting cell

Efferent nerve endings

Afferent nerve endings

Myelin sheath

Figure 3. Structure and innervation of the hair cells. Bending of the cilia of the hair cell occurs due to shift of the gelatinous material that the cilia are embedded in. Deflection causes a polarizing voltage shift across the cell membrane triggering neural impulses within the vestibular nerve.

The second subdivision of the vestibular apparatus is the otoliths. The otoliths include the utricle and saccule (Figure 1) which are platelike structures laden with calcium carbonate crystals, called otoconia, that impart mass to the otolith (Figure 2). Consequently, unlike the semicircular canals, otoliths are sensitive to gravitational and linear acceleration forces in the vertical, lateral, and fore-aft directions.

The receptor cell of the vestibular labyrinth is the hair cell. The vestibular receptor cells are located within the maculae of the utricle and saccule and within the crista ampullaris of the semicircular canals (Figure 2). Hair cells have bundles of cilia which project outwards, and neural activity is either enhanced or suppressed by the bending of these cilia as a consequence of an accelerating motion (Figure 3).

Vestibular pathways

Vestibular afferent information from receptor hair cells is transmitted via the vestibulocochlear or VIII cranial nerve. The cell bodies of the vestibular nerve lie in Scarpa's ganglion, which is situated within the internal auditory canal. Vestibular information then arrives at the brainstem vestibular nuclei. All vestibular afferents are excitatory. Central axons bifurcate into an ascending branch which extends to the superior vestibular nucleus and the cerebellum and a descending branch which reaches the medial, inferior and lateral vestibular nuclei. Most axons concerned with eye movement terminate in the rostral part of the medial nucleus and the superior nucleus.[2]

Vestibular integration
a. The vestibulo-ocular reflex
Within the vestibular nuclei, most second-order afferents are monosynaptic and receive direct input. While some second-order afferents are sensitive purely to head movement, most are affected by eye movement as well. For example, PVP neurons are sensitive to eye position and head velocity, as well as saccadic pauses.[2] Also, Scudder and Fuchs described eye velocity-head velocity neurons as being part of the pathways, which allow vision to either override or enhance vestibular information.[3]

Each semicircular canal has major neural connections to one ipsilateral and one contralateral extraocular muscle. This three- neuron pathway is the basis of the vestibulo-ocular reflex. Within the brainstem, several major tracts carry neural input between the corresponding agonist muscles of the two eyes. For example, the medial longitudinal fasciculus (MLF) and the ascending tract of Deiters (ATD) complete the three-neuron pathway that subserves horizontal conjugate eye movement by connecting the corresponding ipsilateral vestibular nuclei with the contralateral abducens nucleus and lateral rectus to the ipsilateral oculomotor nucleus and medial rectus.

The vestibulo-ocular reflex (VOR) adds to the maintenance of foveal fixation during head movement. Since the three pairs of semicircular canals represent all rotational movements in three-dimensional space, vision will be maintained for all directions of head movement. In addition to the excitatory pathway described above, second-order inhibitory neurons will innervate the corresponding antagonist eye muscles.

b. Postural control
Vestibulospinal pathways also arise from the vestibular nuclei in the brainstem. The lateral and medial vestibulospinal tracts carry vestibular information from the lateral and medial vestibular nuclei, respectively, to the anterior horn cells of the spinal cord. The vestibulospinal reflexes are directly responsible for postural control under static and dynamic conditions. Generally, the lateral tract influences extensor muscles of the lower limbs

and trunk, while the medial tract influences reflex head and upper torso movements.

c. Motor control
Vestibulocerebellar pathways provide a bidirectional conduit between the flocculonodulus of the cerebellum and the lateral vestibular nuclei. These pathways serve a modulating function of motor output and act as integrators of motor activity.

d. Cortical sites
At the cerebral level, animal studies[4-6] have identified several regions within the parietal and temporal lobes which receive afferent vestibular information. Through electrode stimulation studies,[7,8] PET imaging,[9-11] and functional MRI[12,13] in humans, it has become evident that unlike other sensory modalities such as vision and somatosensation, there is no primary vestibular cortex. Rather, vestibular afferent information appears to be transmitted to association cortex regions, which also receive afferent input from primary and secondary visual, and to lesser degree, somatosensory centers. Interestingly, these vestibular regions have cytotechtonic architecture that is more typical of multisensory cortex than primary sensory cortex.

It appears that the parietoinsular cortex is a major site of vestibular projections. Half of the neurons in this region respond to vestibular information. However, in keeping with the concept of a multisensory cortex, neurons in this region also respond to visual optokinetic and somatosensory stimulation.[14] Thus, the parietoinsular cortical region appears to be involved in the processing and integration of visual, vestibular and somatosensory information.

This integration of multisensory information involves an inhibitory reciprocal process in which activation of vestibular pathways results in inhibition of visual information and vice versa. The functional significance of this inhibitory reciprocal sensory interaction is immediately clear in traumatic brain injury. This mechanism allows a potential mismatch between two conflicting sensory inputs to be suppressed by shifting the sensorial weight to the dominant modality.[12] It is logical that the traumatized brain, which has lost this capacity, will be unable to reconcile visual, vestibular and somatosensory conflict, resulting in balance instability and dizziness.

The visual system
The visual system is the second major component of the afferent-efferent model relating to balance. As discussed previously, the vestibular nucleus receives visual, somatosensory and auditory input. In association with the

VOR, it is important for maintaining a stable visual-spatial world when head and body movements are involved.

The peripheral visual component

Similar to the vestibular system, the visual system has both peripheral and central components. The peripheral component essentially gathers photoptic information and converts this information to electrical energy. It comprises the eye itself, along with the extraocular muscles, accommodative system and the optical media.

Although diplopia is an obvious cause of visual confusion related to the dysfunction of the peripheral component, clinical experience has shown that more subtle visual and oculomotor dysfunctions are commonly associated with vestibular symptoms. For example, as discussed earlier in this chapter, the VOR is dependent on a stable bifoveal retinal image. Thus, uncompensated binocular deviations such as fixation disparity, phoria, convergence insufficiency, and accommodative convergence dysfunctions are commonly associated with symptoms of vestibular dysfunction. In a broad sense, any mismatch of visual information could potentially exacerbate a vestibular problem. Many patients have moderate vertical and horizontal phorias that may have been well compensated for most of their lives. However, an illness or other stress factor can result in a breakdown of fusional control; the decompensation of binocularity can add to the mismatching of afferent information affecting the VOR and ultimately balance.

The central visual component

The central aspect of this process is organized through two main and separate systems. These were first identified as focal and ambient. Subsequent research further specified these systems as parvocellular (P) and magnocellular (M), respectively. Table 1 compares their characteristics. These systems are defined by their retinal elements, pathways and specific functions.

The P-system is for central foveal vision and is important for clear and precise form vision. These nerve fibers start at the retina and travel via the optic nerve, the optic chiasm and optic tract to synapse at the lateral geniculate nucleus. They then proceed to the optic radiations, to the primary visual cortex in the occipital lobes and then to the temporal brain region.

The M-system primarily provides general spatial orientation and information. It contributes to balance, movement, coordination and posture. Some of these fibers from the peripheral retina, which are part of the ambient visual system, are directed primarily to the midbrain and synapse at the lat-

Table 1. Characteristics of Magnocellular and Parvocellular Subsystems	
Magnocellular	Parvocellular
1. Most sensitive to low and middle spatial frequencies: large overall shapes.	1. Most sensitive to high spatial frequencies: fine detail.
2. High sensitivity to contrast.	2. Low sensitivity to contrast.
3. Peripheral vision dominant.	3. Central (foveal) vision dominant.
4. Responds to onset and offset of stimulus. Short response persistence (transient).	4. Responds during and after stimulus presentation. Longer response persistence.
5. Most sensitive to high temporal frequencies.	5. Most sensitive to low temporal frequencies.
6. Responds quickly to moving targets (early warning).	6. Sensitive to stationary or slowly-moving targets.
7. Sensitive to short wavelengths (e.g., blue).	7. Sensitive to longer wavelengths (e.g., red).
8. Global analysis of incoming visual information.	8. Identification of shapes and patterns.
9. Involved in perception of depth, flicker, motion, brightness, discrimination.	9. Involved in processing color information.
10. Prepares visual system for the input of slower detailed information that follows.	10. Responds subsequent to transient output and is dependent upon transient output.

Reprinted with permission from the Journal of Behavioral Optometry. Solan HA. Transient and sustained processing: a dual subsystem theory of reading disability. 1994;5(6):151.

eral geniculate body and then the superior colliculus, which is important for integrating posture, movement, and orientation to positional space. Other fibers continue to the occipital cortex, and then to the temporal and parietal brain areas.

The superior colliculus receives visual, auditory and somatosensory stimuli and is involved in reflex turning of the head towards the source of the stimuli. Visual information originates both directly from the eyes as well as the visual cortex. Auditory and somatosensory stimuli reach the superior colliculus via projections from the inferior colliculus and spinal cord, respectively. Since the superior colliculus receives fibers from the optic tract, occipital cortex and spinotectal tract, it becomes linked with the kinesthetic, proprioceptive, vestibular and tactile systems.

Thus, the ambient visual system (M-system) is important in providing information about where one is in space and where one is looking, while the focal system (P-system) provides information about the details of the object of regard. Finally, appropriately coordinated head and body postural reflexes are generated as information flows across the vestibulocerebellar and vestibulospinal tracts. [15-19]

Vestibular signals that are produced as a consequence of reflex head movements (i.e., VOR) are evaluated by integrating mechanisms and rendered inappropriate. The suppression of the VOR reflex allows the generation of appropriate saccade and pursuit eye movements. An application of this principle has given rise to a "substitution" exercise strategy used during vestibular rehabilitation called VOR cancellation. If this did not occur, then the mismatching of visual information with other elements of the sensorimotor feedback system could cause one to perceive an image as jumping and moving with shift of gaze.

The somatosensory system

The somatosensory system is the third and final component of the afferent-efferent model of balance. Detection of position begins with mechanoreceptors located within the skin, joints and muscles. Primary afferent somatosensory information is then carried within the peripheral nervous system along large myelinated fibers whose neuronal bodies reside within the dorsal root ganglia of the spinal cord. Proximal transmission then continues via the posterior or dorsal columns of the spinal cord. Second-order neurons within the nucleus gracilis and nucleus cuneatus then cross contralaterally via the medial lemniscus to the thalamus. Processing and integration of somatosensory information takes place at this level and is then further transmitted to primary somatosensory cortex within the parietal lobe as well as to the cerebellum. Further processing of somatosensory information takes place at this level. Final processing within secondary and association cortex within the parietal, frontal, and temporal lobes with integrated motor responses from the cerebellum occurs. As previously discussed, it is at this level that multisensory integration as well as conscious perception takes place.

An Integrated Model of Balance

A more sophisticated model of balance now emerges. At the most basic level is reception. The neuroanatomic substrates of the afferent system have already been discussed. The process of integration, which has already been touched upon, occurs at several levels of the neurosensory pathways. For example, the first stage of vestibular processing takes place within the vestibular nuclei of the brainstem. Reciprocal neural pathways between the vestibular nuclei, thalamus and cerebellum clearly result in information processing. It is likely that at the level of the thalamus and cerebellum, the first integration and processing of parallel information from the visual, vestibular and somatosensory systems occurs.

Further and final integration of sensory information takes place within the cerebrum. The primary visual cortex and the primary somatosensory cortex process information, which is then integrated with information from secondary and association cortical regions.

It appears that conscious perception of sensation takes place at this highest level. Sensory conflict or mismatch, which may take place at any stage along the sensory pathway, is perceived only when all information has been processed and integrated within these cortical regions. The inability to reconcile any conflict will result in the perception of vertigo, dizziness and imbalance.

Further involvement of cognitive/intellectual and psychological processes has an overwhelming "coloring" effect on the perception and consequences of these rudimentary sensory conflicts.

Two additional concepts must be introduced into the framework of vestibular physiology. In considering the overall functionality of the vestibular system in particular and the balance system in toto, the multiple layering of information processing and motor responses becomes evident. This arrangement provides several advantages. First, the parallel processing of information by its nature requires a reconciliation of different sensory inputs, which improves the accuracy of the system. Second, redundant information allows a framework for "learning" which can act as a substitute for actual information in situations where information may be lacking or is inaccurate. Finally, redundancy allows for the existence of a plastic and adaptable system that can change, repair and compensate. It is the existence of a redundant and plastic balance system that allows for the success of vestibular, visual, and balance rehabilitation therapy.

Diagnostic Vestibular Testing

Formal evaluation of the vestibular system is often necessary to appreciate fully the underlying physiologic deficits that lead to patient symptoms. A battery of vestibular function tests is often performed. These might include MRI of the brain and internal auditory canals, audiometry, electronystagmography, VOR testing (rotatory chair or vestibular autorotation testing), brainstem auditory evoked responses, and computerized dynamic posturography. In the section that follows, several of these diagnostic modalities are briefly discussed to facilitate an understanding of a typical vestibular evaluation.

Electronystagmography (ENG)

Traditional eye movement recordings take advantage of the eyeball as a dipole. Therefore, eye movements create a voltage differential that can be recorded with electrodes placed around the eyes. However, this method is limited in its ability to record only horizontal and vertical conjugate eye movement.

ENG consists of a battery of tests that include sinusoidal tracking (smooth pursuit), horizontal and vertical gaze testing, saccade eye movements, optokinetic nystagmus testing, position-induced nystagmus testing (supine, head left, and head right directions), the Dix-Hallpike maneuver, and bithermal caloric testing.

The Dix-Hallpike maneuver is performed by recording the provocation of nystagmus as a result of rapid positioning of the head into a left or right hanging position. It is specifically designed to diagnose the presence of benign paroxysmal positional vertigo, which is one of the most common and readily treatable vestibular disorders.

Bithermal caloric testing involves the introduction of cool ($30^{o}C$) or warm ($44^{o}C$) water or air into the external auditory canal. This causes a vector flow of endolymph within the horizontal semicircular canal, thereby inducing nystagmus. Stimulating the same ear above and below body temperature produces nystagmus in different directions. This has been termed COWS (Cold Opposite, Warm Same). The intensity and direction of the nystagmus is compared between each ear to determine the presence of peripheral vestibular dysfunction.

Computerized dynamic posturography (CDP)

Computerized dynamic posturography, commercially known as the Equitest,[a] is designed to assess patients with gait and balance disturbances. Through analysis of changing visual and somatic stimuli, both the sensory (afferent) and motor (efferent) systems necessary for maintenance of balance and posture can be assessed. This is a test of functional integrity and does not provide specific etiologic information. As such, it is unique in the battery of balance testing. It also has a role in the treatment of the dizzy patient. Specific dysfunctions can be determined and appropriate rehabilitation strategies can be initiated.

The Sensory Organization Test component incorporates six testing conditions to analyze the role of somatic, visual and vestibular input into central nervous system interpretation of special orientation (sensory analysis). Additional information about the patient's center of gravity and the use of corrective postural ankle and hip movement is also obtained.

The Motor Control Test component incorporates anterior-posterior and up-down translation of the standing surface to assess for latency, strength, and symmetry of corrective postural responses; weight symmetry; and postural reflex adaptation. This is done through computer analysis of body sway, postural alignment, and sheer forces of the feet against the translating standing surface.

While the Equitest provides quantified and computerized interpretation of test data, similar qualitative information is often obtained with standard "bedside" testing performed by the vestibular therapist.

Vestibular autorotation testing (VAT)

The VAT[b] is another commercially available vestibular test which complements the information provided by ENG. It provides specific diagnostic information about the functional integrity of the vertical and horizontal vestibulo-ocular reflex (VOR). While it does not provide etiologic or localizing disease-specific information, like CDP, the functional information is instrumental in developing appropriate vestibular rehabilitation strategies. Alternatively, several standard "bedside" clinical assessment techniques can provide qualitative information about the integrity of the VOR system.

During the VAT, the patient is seated in a chair and fixates on a target. The patient then rotates his/her head horizontally or vertically in response to a computer-generated tone that increases in frequency from 0.5 Hz to 6.0 Hz. Standard electro-oculography (EOG) electrodes record eye movements while a rotational velocity sensor fastened to a head strap monitors head motion.

Head and eye movements are compared. Data on gain, phase and asymmetry are then analyzed by computer and compared with normative data for final analysis and interpretation.

Brainstem auditory evoked responses (BAER)

Following a series of repeated acoustic stimuli, specific electrical potentials can be recorded from the scalp. Five or more potentials are evoked within the vestibulocochlear nerve and central auditory pathways. These potentials have very specific latencies, and either the delay or absence of these evoked responses signify a localizable dysfunction within the auditory pathway.

This technique is useful in assessing hearing in young or uncooperative patients. Its localizing properties often help in determining possible causes of hearing and vestibular dysfunction. Today, MRI has proven more sensitive and specific than BAER and is now the study of choice in most cases.

Rehabilitation Strategies
Optometric rehabilitation

The Neuro-Optometric Rehabilitation Association (NORA) defines neuro-optometric rehabilitation as the blending of the profession's primary eye and vision care, and the art and science of optometry and vision rehabilitation, to develop an individualized treatment regimen for individuals with visual deficits as a result of physical disabilities, traumatic brain injuries, and neurological insults and aging. Neuro-optometric therapy is a process for the rehabilitation of functional visual problems as well as visual-perceptual motor disorders. It includes, but is not limited to, acquired strabismus, diplopia, binocular dysfunction, convergence and accommodation problems, versional oculomotor dysfunction, visual-spatial dysfunction, visual-perceptual and cognitive deficits, and traumatic visual acuity loss.[20]

After a neurological event, such as traumatic brain injury, whiplash, multiple sclerosis, cerebrovascular accident, or even the normal aging process, the peripheral and central visual systems may be compromised, which can affect one's ability to match visual information with information from the other components of the sensorimotor loop, often exacerbating vestibular dysfunction. For example, M-system involvement may affect how the ambient process provides information about orientation relative to the patient's true body midline. Often the patient will adjust to this visual mismatch by shifting his/her weight and will actually walk as if the floor is tilted. The rehabilitation optometrist can prescribe yoked prism lenses that help to reestablish visuomotor balance. These lenses in conjunction with physical therapy and optometric visual therapy can positively affect the overall rehabilitative process.[20]

As discussed earlier in this chapter, the brain is a mediator between information from the visual system, vestibular system and proprioceptive system. In a sense, the joints, eyes and ears make up the "keyboard" to the "computer," the brain. The efficiency and accuracy of the brain's software is only as good as the information it receives. The visual problems discussed earlier can be an agent of dissonance, thereby exacerbating the symptoms associated with vestibular and balance problems. The very nature of vestibular treatment modalities often is dependent on stable visual information. Thus, in many cases, eliminating the visual problem is often the key to significant progress in vestibular rehabilitation, while at other times, treating the vestibular dysfunction enhances gains in vision therapy.

Vestibular rehabilitation

Vestibular rehabilitation is an exercise-based approach to the treatment of persons with vestibular dysfunction. The use of exercise for treatment of this population is well documented.[21,22]

Description of all vestibular disease presentations that can be helped by exercise-based rehabilitation is beyond the scope of this chapter. Therefore, we will briefly describe the common complaints that pertain to the clinical cases to be presented later.

Because of its connection with the visual system, somatosensory system and cortex, dysfunction of the vestibular system can cause difficulties maintaining foveal fixation, postural control and movement.

As defined earlier, the VOR adds to the maintenance of foveal fixation during head movement. In rehabilitation, this is referred to as gaze stabilization.

VOR dysfunction causes retinal slip. This occurs when incorrect neuronal input from the vestibular system to the eye muscles does not allow the eyes to maintain a stable image on the retina. Vestibular rehabilitation uses co-ordinated head and eye movements to facilitate central adaptation and/or substitution of other sensory input mechanisms. Central adaptation occurs as the brain attempts to correct the abnormal neuronal input it is receiving from the dysfunctional vestibular system by centrally adjusting the effective VOR gain. Substitution for lost vestibular function uses sensory inputs from the cervico-ocular reflex, as well as smooth pursuit and saccadic eye movements.[23,24]

Vestibulospinal reflex dysfunction creates postural instabilities that become more pronounced during movement or in challenging sensory environments (e.g., dimly lit areas, uneven surfaces). Recovery of postural stability can occur through central adaptation and/or substitution. As with the VOR, the brain adjusts the vestibular spinal responses in the attempt to minimize postural instability. Rehabilitation may also encourage the use of visual and somatosensory information instead of the erroneous vestibular information. Static balance is defined as the ability to maintain an upright posture during nonmovement positioning. Dynamic balance is the ability to maintain upright posture during movement due to either internal or external perturbation.

Patients suffering from vestibular dysfunction are often sensitive to motion. Habituation exercises involve repetitive movements to desensitize the central nervous system.[25]

Case Illustrations

The following cases illustrate the importance of a multidisciplinary approach to the management of patients who have balance and vestibular disorders. Each case will review the major symptoms and key diagnostic information provided by the neurologist, optometrist and physical therapist. This will be followed by an overview of the optometric and physical therapy treatment plans and patient outcome.

Case 1
Neurotologic evaluation
A 78-year-old woman complained of episodic vertigo and nausea for 18 years. Additionally, for the past six months, she had had constant imbalance resulting in occasional falls. One fall caused a minor closed-head injury without loss of consciousness. She denied tinnitus, weakness or numbness.

The patient had a history of diabetes, hypertension, chronic cough, and arthritis, for which she took lisinopril, hydrochlorothiazide, metoprolol, diltiazem hydrochloride, and metformin hydrochloride. Her surgical history included cholecystectomy, right stapes surgery 35 years previously, and two left ear surgeries with the latest for hearing loss. She had bilateral iridectomy for cataracts.

She was afebrile with a blood pressure of 145 systolic, a pulse of 80, and respirations of 16. The remainder of the general examination was unremarkable except for mild restricted mobility of the neck and right shoulder.

Neurological examination was unremarkable except for a wide unsteady gait with spontaneous retropulsion. She was not able to tandem walk or perform either the Romberg Test or Fekuda Marching Test. Additionally, there was diminished sensation in the distal lower extremities.

Otology examination was notable for a right hearing aid. Hearing was reduced bilaterally, especially on the left, with bone conduction greater than air conduction to a 128 Hz tuning fork. The tympanic membrane was dull on the right. There was a small perforation on the left.

Her neurological eye examination revealed full visual fields and a normal funduscopic examination. The pupils were irregular due to previous iridectomy. Extraocular movements were normal.

MRI of the brain revealed diffuse atrophy. Left caloric weakness indicating left peripheral vestibular dysfunction was seen on electronystagmography. Brainstem auditory evoked response test showed severe bilateral hearing loss. Vestibular autorotation test was normal. Balance abnormalities due to vestibular and visual dysfunction, poor adaptation and inappropriate ankle strategy were demonstrated on computerized dynamic posturography.

Physical therapy evaluation
Dizziness, gaze stability, static and dynamic balance and motion sensitivity were evaluated.

I- Subjective Reports
Scored 80 out of 100 on the Dizziness Handicap Inventory (100 being worst perceived symptomatology).

II- Gaze Stability
Corrective saccades were demonstrated with mild undershooting during horizontal and vertical smooth pursuit testing. There was no spontaneous or gaze-evoked nystagmus noted.

Head thrust test was not performed because of neck stiffness.

During convergence screening, the nearpoint was markedly receded at 12 inches with diplopia.

Frenzel lens examination revealed no spontaneous or gaze-evoked nystagmus; however, a minimal clockwise and downbeat nystagmus was noted following head shaking side to side. The Frenzel lens device consists of a high-powered convex lenses (+20D) and an illumination system in a special goggle worn by the patient. When this system is placed on the patient in reduced room illumination, nystagmus is easily observed under this very blurred visual condition that does not permit fixation to take place.

Able to read with correction OD 20/20 (-1), OS 20/25. Binocularly, with head oscillations of 2 Hz the patient attained 20/40 but reported diplopia.

III- Static and Dynamic Balance
Performed modified Romberg Test (feet positioned 12 inches apart) eyes open/eyes closed for 60 out of expected 60 seconds. Unable to perform standard Romberg Test eyes open/eyes closed.

Able to ambulate with wide base of support and upper extremity guarding but requiring 28 seconds for 75 feet of ambulation, thus necessitating close supervision. Required 35 seconds for 75 feet of ambulation turning head left and center every three steps and required contact guard/minimal assistance.

IV- Motion Sensitivity
Did not tolerate motion sensitivity testing. No nystagmus was evident during bilateral modified Dix-Hallpike maneuvers despite complaints of a severe increase in symptoms.

V- Computerized Binocular Vision Screening
Failed in the areas of fusional, saccadic and pursuit testing, and demonstrated a significant fixation disparity. Consequently, she was referred for a rehabilitative optometric evaluation.

Summary

Diagnostic tests as well as clinical evaluation suggested vestibulopathy with severe positional sensitivity present. Static and dynamic balance deficits were a result of a combination of vestibular, neuropathic and oculomotor dysfunction, which affected the visual balance system. Convergence screening and results of visual acuity testing further suggested an associated visual dysfunction. Consequently, balance complaints were thought to be multifactorial in etiology. This included peripheral vestibular dysfunction, hearing loss, visual impairment, sensory loss due to diabetic polyneuropathy, and mechanical dysfunction due to arthritis.

Optometric evaluation

After reviewing the medical and vision history, the evaluation focused on the patient's symptoms as they related to the balance problems. For the past two to three years, she had experienced diplopia with variable separation associated with compensatory head movement. She could not sustain reading because the words appeared to move and blur. She also had difficulty judging depth, especially with curbs and stairs.

I- Ocular health was unremarkable except for bilateral pseudoaphakia with posterior chamber intraocular lenses (IOL) in each eye.

II- Refractive analysis revealed:
OD –0.25-1.25x90 20/20(-2), OS –0.50-1.00x60 20/25(-1).

Nearpoint testing indicated a +3.00 add which provided vision of 20/20 from 10 inches to 15 inches.

III- Sensorimotor exam revealed a moderate esophoria at distance with inadequate fusional ranges and intermittent diplopia. With 3 prism diopters base-out, she was able to exhibit fusion. Near testing through the indicated prescription revealed esophoria, with inadequate compensating fusion ranges and a receded nearpoint of convergence of 8 inches with recovery at 12 inches.

Summary

Poorly compensated convergence excess with secondary convergence insufficiency resulting in unstable visual input to the vestibular system.

Rehabilitation management
Vestibular rehabilitation

Over three months, the patient was instructed in static and dynamic balance exercises and habituation exercises that were performed in the clinic and as a daily home exercise program. Vestibulo-ocular reflex exercises were deferred until further evaluation of the oculomotor status.

Optometric management
The patient's lens prescription was changed from a progressive addition type to separate distance and near prescriptions. A total of five prism diopters, equally divided between the two lenses, was incorporated into the prescriptions. Optometric vision therapy to improve oculomotor control, as well as to increase fusional stability and normalize convergence range was initiated. The first phase of the treatment program focused on the enhancement of oculomotor control under stressful balance and visual conditions. Thus, the patient was positioned on a balance board and wore yoked prisms. She was instructed to fixate a light directly in front of her. When aware of a peripheral lighted target, she was required to fixate that target and accurately locate it with a handheld laser pointer. This technique first requires a reorganization of visual information as a result of the yoked prisms and then an integration of this information with vestibular and proprioceptive inputs, which should result in an accurate motor response. During the second phase of treatment, fusional facility was increased at all distances with the ultimate goal of maintaining flat fusion and fusional recovery (divergence and convergence). The final phase incorporated tasks that required the patient to maintain balance while she alternately converged and diverged her eyes. The patient completed 16 sessions of vision therapy.

Summary of all treatment results
Gaze stability
With the new lenses, she was able to read 20/20 OU and 20/40 OU with head rotation at 2 Hz, and she no longer complained of diplopia.

Static and dynamic balance
She was able to perform half-sharpened Romberg Test eyes open/eyes closed 60 out of expected 60 seconds. This was a significant improvement from the initial evaluation.

She was able to ambulate moving her head right and left every two steps for 75 feet thus demonstrating minimal loss of balance.

Motion sensitivity
Her motion sensitivity was within normal limits, and she no longer demonstrated positional symptomatology.

The patient reported that she was now able to read comfortably for prolonged periods and that her depth judgment was significantly improved. Most of her balance difficulty on stairs and curbs had resolved.

The patient scored 12 out of 100 on the Dizziness Handicap Inventory, thus demonstrating a significant improvement from her initial score of 80.

Case 2
Neurotologic evaluation

A 65-year-old man presented for neurological assessment of seizures. A previous neurological evaluation included a brain MRI that was normal, an EEG that did not show seizure activity, and an unremarkable cardiac evaluation. He was treated with Dilantin. He also complained of episodes of dizziness and a drunken feeling with loss of balance when bending over. Postural movements provoked these episodes. They predated the use of Dilantin. Tinnitus, hearing loss and nausea were present.

The patient had no significant past medical history. He was taking no other medications and denied alcohol abuse.

Blood pressure was 120/80 mm Hg with a normal pulse. Neurological examination was unremarkable except for mild bilateral gaze-evoked nystagmus, which could be a side effect of Dilantin. His gait was slightly wide-based with some difficulty performing tandem walking. Otological examination found the tympanic membranes to be clear. Hearing was normal. His neurological eye examination revealed full eye movements, normal visual fields and normal pupils (equal, round and reactive).

Diagnostic evaluation of his dizziness included a normal brain MRI and BAER. Electronystagmography revealed poor vertical smooth pursuit of central etiology as well as right-beating nystagmus during the head hanging right Dix-Hallpike maneuver. VAT revealed decreased horizontal responses. Consequently, the patient was referred for vestibular rehabilitation therapy.

Physical therapy evaluation

I- Subjective

The patient scored a 46 out of 100 on the Dizziness Handicap Inventory (100 being worst perceived symptomatology).

II- Gross Musculoskeletal and Neurological Evaluation

Musculoskeletal evaluation revealed moderate limitations in active range of motion of the cervical spine. Gross neurological evaluation was unremarkable for upper and lower extremity coordination, strength and sensation.

III- Gaze Stabilization

Gaze stability evaluation suggested deficits in binocular vision, with the patient reporting diplopia at 10 inches during gross convergence screening. Dynamic gaze stability deficits were noted with the VOR assessment at 2Hz. A right-beating spontaneous nystagmus with Fresnel lenses and a down-beating nystagmus following head shaking side to side with Fresnel lenses were seen as well, with both further implying vestibular dysfunction.

IV- Static and Dynamic Balance

Balance evaluation demonstrated static deficits. The patient was able to perform half-sharpened Romberg Test with right head tilt for 60 out of expected 60 seconds and with left head tilt 30 out of expected 60 seconds. The patient turned 90° to the left during the Fekuda Marching Test in place. The patient was increasingly symptomatic during ambulation with turning head right and left every three steps.

V- Motion Sensitivity

Position sensitivity assessment utilizing the Motion Sensitivity Test indicated minimal positional sensitivity.

Summary

This patient demonstrated VOR dysfunction with only minor static balance deficits and positional sensitivity. Convergence insufficiency could limit the effectiveness of vestibular rehabilitation, and therefore the patient was referred for neuro-optometric assessment and treatment.

Optometric evaluation

The patient's past eye and medical histories were reviewed. The patient's primary visual symptom was intermittent and variable diplopia over the past two years. He reported diplopia when playing golf, driving, reading and performing his work as a sculptor. He experienced significant symptoms of lightheadedness and the sensation that his space world was "swimming," which became more pronounced when he was in a complex and moving visual environment. Additionally, he often perceived that the floor was tilted and moving, and he had difficulty judging depth accurately.

I- Eye health evaluation: essentially normal with mild crystalline lens changes consistent with his age.

II- Refractive analysis:

OD +3.00 20/20, OS +3.75-0.25x165 20/25+ and a reading add of +2.50.

III- Sensorimotor examination revealed a noncomitant deviation. At distance, he manifested right hyperesotropia. The angle of deviation was variable, with the vertical component increasing in superior and left gaze. At near with his reading lenses, he manifested an intermittent exotropia with a variable right hypertropia which decreased in down gaze. He had an extremely receded nearpoint of convergence of 12 inches with fusional recovery at 16 inches. The Park 3-Step revealed left superior rectus involvement. Further, there was a mild abduction restriction of the right eye. He showed a compensatory head tilt up and to the left.

Rehabilitation Management
Vestibular rehabilitation
The vestibulo-ocular reflex exercise using full-field focus produced an increase in overall symptoms and complaints of diplopia during the exercise. Performance of the half-sharpened Romberg Test with head tilt improved. The patient continued to demonstrate a 90° turn to the left during the Fekuda Marching Test. The Motion Sensitivity Test score improved.

The patient experienced only slight improvement despite one month of intensive therapy. While improvements were noted in motion sensitivity, he was not responding to traditional vestibular rehabilitation with respect to his dynamic gaze stability. Although the positional dizziness had resolved, he noted residual dizziness during reading, as well as when gazing up or down or when changing his viewing distance. He felt most of his symptoms to be visually related. He once again scored 46 out of 100 on the Dizziness Handicap Inventory. Accordingly, neuro-optometric evaluation was advised.

Optometric management
The patient's spectacles were changed from progressive addition lenses to individual distance and near lenses. Vertical prism to compensate for the hypertropic deviation was incorporated into both spectacles. The goals of orthoptic visual therapy were to enhance oculomotor control and to develop adequate fusional facility and recovery, especially during head and eye movements.

To stabilize the vertical component of the ocular deviation, vertical prisms were prescribed. The first phase of treatment stressed the improvement of oculomotor control using prisms to expand the range of abduction. Additionally, sequences were initially added to increase fusional ability in space, especially at his centration point, and eventually with head movement and variation in gaze direction. The final phase incorporated therapy sequences which required flat fusion and speed of fusional recovery with head and body movement.

With his spectacles, he demonstrated excellent fusional control in all positions of gaze and a normal convergence nearpoint. He reported that his visual symptoms were eliminated and that he was now able to play golf and sculpt without difficulty. His dizziness and lightheadedness were significantly reduced.

Case 3
Neurotologic evaluation
A 48-year-old woman presented with a two-year history of dizziness without vertigo. There was a rocking, seasick feeling with nausea and loss of balance that was worsened by head motion but not by specific position. The symptoms were continuous and lasted weeks. There was no tinnitus, hearing loss, or headache. ENT and ophthalmologic evaluations were normal.

Past medical history included depression and sinus allergies. Her medications included Triphasil 21, Wellbutrin, and Vancenase. She denied alcohol use.

Clinical examination revealed a blood pressure of 125/70 with a normal pulse. Neurological examination was normal. Neurotological examination revealed nystagmus on left gaze during the left Dix-Hallpike maneuver. She turned to the left during the marching test and had difficulty with tandem walking. Hearing was normal. Her pupils were equal and reactive. Visual fields were full to confrontation.

Diagnostic testing included a normal brain MRI and BAER. ENG revealed left-beating nystagmus in the head left position. VAT found a weak horizontal response.

Accordingly, the patient was referred for vestibular rehabilitation therapy.

Physical therapy evaluation
Medical history, previous clinical examinations and diagnostic test results were reviewed. Gaze stability, static and dynamic balance and motion sensitivity were evaluated.

I- Subjective Complaints
   The patient scored 58 out of 100 on the Dizziness Handicap Inventory (100 is worst perceived symptomatology) and 42 out of 99 on the Functional Check List (99 is worst perceived functional limitations).

II- Gaze Stability
   Smooth pursuit and saccadic testing were normal. No spontaneous or gaze-evoked nystagmus was noted. Fresnel lens examination demonstrated no spontaneous or gaze-evoked nystagmus. There was minimal down-beating nystagmus following head shaking from side to side. Head thrust test was normal. During convergence testing, the patient reported diplopia.
   During dynamic visual acuity testing the patient was able to read 20/20 OS, 20/20 OD, 20/20 OU and 20/25 OU with head rotation of 2 Hz,

with the reduction of visual acuity indicating VOR gaze stability difficulty.

III- Static and Dynamic Balance

The patient was able to perform half-sharpened Romberg Test eyes open/eyes closed. She complained of unsteadiness and dizziness with ambulation with head turning right and left every two steps.

IV- Motion Sensitivity

The patient scored 20%, which indicated moderate to severe positional sensitivity.

Summary

Diagnostic tests and clinical evaluation suggested peripheral vestibulopathy with positional component. The patient continued with a home vestibular and general conditioning exercise program.

Optometric evaluation

Her past medical and ocular history was reviewed. She was a computer graphics artist who had been experiencing vestibular problems for the past two years. Specifically, she felt "out of balance" with her space world, which increased if she fixated on an object straight ahead. She experienced a feeling of lightheadedness when driving, reading and working on her computer. Additionally, the lightheadedness increased when she changed her fixation from the computer to distance and back to the computer.

I- Ocular health examination was normal.

II- Refractive analysis revealed:
OD+0.25 20/20, OS+0.25 20/20, and a +2.50 reading addition.

III- Sensorimotor exam revealed orthophoria at distance and an intermittent exotropia at near with a significantly reduced nearpoint of convergence to 12 inches. Fusional ranges at nearpoint were characteristic of a convergence insufficiency with the need for base-in prism to fuse.

Rehabilitation management

Vestibular rehabilitation

The patient was given exercises at the clinic as well as a daily home exercise program. Exercises emphasized vestibulo-ocular reflex training, habituation exercises for her positional symptoms and general conditioning. At her two-month reevaluation, she complained of difficulty with night vision and focusing during computer work. A binocular vision screening was performed. The patient failed in the area of fusional ranges and manifested an intermittent left exotropia. A formal neuro-optometric evaluation was recommended.

Optometric management

Bifocal lenses were prescribed with one prescription for her working distance for the monitor and one for reading and close work, with both incorporating a computer tint. She completed 15 visits of vision therapy for convergence insufficiency, which eliminated all of her visual symptoms.

Summary of treatment results

I- Subjective

Reported significant improvement in symptoms. She scored a 12 out of 100 on the Dizziness Handicap Inventory and 3 out of 99 on the Functional Checklist, both significant improvements from the initial evaluation. She continued to complain of difficulty with night vision and focusing on the computer.

II- Gaze Stability

Read 20/20 OU and 20/20 OU with head rotations at 2 Hz.

III- Static and Dynamic Balance

Able to perform half-sharpened Romberg Test eyes open/eyes closed with little if any demonstration of sway.

Able to walk on a treadmill at 2.2–2.5 mph for 20 minutes with head turns right and left every two steps for four 30-second intervals with no significant demonstration of sway and no complaints of increase in symptoms.

IV- Motion Sensitivity

Score 0% on the motion sensitivity test, which is a significant improvement from the initial evaluation.

Conclusion

Dizziness, balance problems, and vertigo (the sensation that the spatial world is moving) are some of the most commonly reported problems in general medical practice. Vestibular function is important for the maintenance of balance and a stable visual environment. Persons with central nervous system injury, other idiopathic causes of visual processing problems, or functional vision problems that are not adequately managed, often experience extreme difficulty with balance and movement, as well as with their perception of visual space. Since vestibular rehabilitation therapy requires the presence of an intact visual system, it is understandable that such patients will experience limited therapeutic benefit. Consequently, patients often experience difficulty functioning in environments with excessive visual stimulation, such as grocery stores or shopping malls. Often movement in a crowded environment becomes quite disturbing and causes vertiginous symptoms.

Successful balance and movement is the outcome of the integration of information from the vestibular, visual and somatosensory systems. The integration of this information takes place at multiple levels within the central nervous system from the brainstem through the cerebral cortex. This process is both plastic and redundant. Consequently, there is a great capacity for recovery following injury to the central nervous system.

Visual and vestibular rehabilitation takes advantage of this concept. Initial attempts at vestibular rehabilitation therapy of individuals with central nervous system injury are often met with incomplete responses. In the past few years, it has become apparent that a comprehensive multidisciplinary approach combining visual and vestibular therapy yields the greatest therapeutic benefit. The first case presented illustrates this multidisciplinary approach. While the patient clearly had vestibular deficits, there was only a partial response to vestibular rehabilitation therapy. When therapeutic attention was directed towards the patient's visual deficits, significant progress was made. Only after a multidisciplinary approach was undertaken, combining both vestibular and visual rehabilitation techniques, was there a successful therapeutic outcome. Clearly, disciplinary-specific therapeutic strategies in isolation were ineffective.

Often patients with significant visual and visual-motor dysfunction have symptoms which suggest an underlying vestibular dysfunction. This is understandable in the context of the integrating processes that take place within the central nervous system. Certainly persons with head trauma are candidates for such difficulties. Therefore, the vestibular specialist must always consider the possibility of a nonvestibular etiology.

The second patient presented is a good example of such a situation. This patient presented with symptoms and diagnostic test results that implicated vestibular dysfunction as the cause of the dizziness. It was only after vestibular rehabilitation therapy was unsuccessful that a visual etiology was considered and successfully treated.

Finally, many patients with diffuse head trauma manifest symptoms that suggest injury to both the vestibular and visual systems. While the first case illustrated a situation in which correction of the visual dysfunction was necessary to achieve benefit from vestibular rehabilitation therapy, some patients will have non-interactive deficits of both systems. Isolated visual or vestibular therapy will provide benefits within its specific realm. Yet the patient remains dissatisfied. It is only following completion of both therapeutic modalities that the patient achieves significant functional recovery.

In summary, patients with central nervous system injury such as head trauma may experience damage to both visual and vestibular systems causing balance instability and dizziness. Traditional vestibular rehabilitation therapy may provide only a partial remedy. A better understanding of the integrating processes within the central nervous system has cultivated the concept of a multidisciplinary approach in balance therapy. Combining the expertise of the neurotologist and neuro-optometrist provides the highest likelihood of success in the brain-injured patient.

References

1. Hain TC, Hillman MA. Anatomy and physiology of the normal vestibular system. In: Herdman SJ, ed. Vestibular Rehabilitation. Philadelphia: FA Davis, 1994:3-21.

2. Baloh RW, Halmagyi GM. Disorders of the Vestibular System. New York: Oxford University Press, 1996.

3. Scudder CA, Fuchs AF. Physiological and behavioral identification of vestibular nucleus neurons mediating the horizontal vestibulo-ocular reflex in trained rhesus monkeys. J Neurophysiol 1992; 68:244-64.

4. Pandya DN, Sanides F. Architectonic parcellation of the temporal operculum in rhesus monkey and its projection pattern. Z Anat Entwicklungsg 1973; 139:127-61.

5. Walzl EM, Mountcastle VB. Projection of vestibular nerve to cerebral cortex of the cat. Am J Physiol 1949; 159:595-9.

6. Mickle WA, Ades HW. A composite sensory projection area in the cerebral cortex of the cat. Am J Physiol 1952; 170:682-9.

7. Penfield W, Jasper H. Epilepsy and the functional anatomy of the human brain. Boston: Little Brown, 1954.

8. Foerster O. Sensory cortical fields. In: Bumke O, Foerster O eds. Handbook of Neurology. Berlin: Springer, 1936:358-449.

9. Wenzel R, Bartenstein P, Janek A, Dieterich M, Danek A, Weindl A, Minoshima S et al. Deactivation of human visual cortex during involuntary ocular oscillations: a PET activation study. Brain 1996; 119:101-10.

10. Bottini G. Sterzi R, Paulescu E et al. Identification of the central vestibular projections in man: a positron emission tomography activation study. Exp Brain Res 1994; 99:164-9.

11. Brandt T, Bartenstein P, Janek A, Dieterich M. Reciprocal inhibitory vestibular-visual interaction: visual motion stimulation deactivates the parieto-insular vestibular cortex. Brain 1998; 121:1749-58.

12. Dieterich M, Brandt T. Brain activation studies on visual-vestibular and ocular motor interaction. Current Opinions in Neurology 2000 Feb; 13(1):13-8.

13. Bucher SF, Dieterich M, Wiesman M et al. Cerebral functional magnetic resonance imaging of vestibular, auditory, and nociceptive areas during galvanic stimulation. Ann Neurol 1998; 44:120-5.

14. Guldin WO, Grusser OJ. The anatomy of the vestibular cortices of primates. In: Collard M, Jeannerod M, Christen Y, eds. Le Cortex Vestibulaire: Réunion d'Experts, Strasbourg, le 20 Octobre. Paris: Editions Irvinn, 1966:17-26.

15. Skarf B, Glaser JS, Trick LG, Mutlukan E. Neuro ophthalmic exam: the visual system. In: Tasman W, Jaeger E, eds. Duane's Ophthalmology on CD-Rom. Philadelphia: Lippincott, Williams & Wilkins, 2000.

16. Barton J, Barton S, Rizzo M. Visual dysfunctions from lesions of the cerebral cortex. In: Tasman W, Jaeger E, eds. Duane's Ophthalmology on CD-Rom. Philadelphia: Lippincott, Williams & Wilkins, 2000.

17. Miller N, Newman JN, eds. Walsh & Hoyt's Clinical Neuro-Ophthalmology. 5th ed. Baltimore: Williams & Wilkins, 1998.

18. Felleman DV, Van Essen DC. Distributed hierarchical processing in the primate cerebral cortex. Cereb Cortex 1991;1(1):1-47.

19. Kaas, JH. Changing concepts of visual cortex organization in primates. In: Brown JD, ed. Neuropsychology of Visual Perception. Hillsdale NJ: Erlbaum Associates, 1989:3-32.

20. Padula W. Neuro-Optometric Rehabilitation. 3rd ed. Santa Ana, CA: Optometric Extension Program, 2000.

21. Horak FB et al. Effects of vestibular rehabilitation on dizziness and imbalance. Otolaryngol Head Neck Surg 1992 Feb;106(2):175-80.

22. Shepard NT, Telian SA. Programmatic vestibular rehabilitation. Otolaryngol Head Neck Surg 1995 Jan;112(1):173-82.

23. Segal BN, Katsarkas A. Long term deficits of goal-directed vestibulo-ocular function following total unilateral loss of peripheral vestibular function. Acta Otolaryngol (Stockh) 1998 Jul-Aug;106(1-2):102-10.

24. Leigh RJ et al. Supplementation of the vestibulo-ocular reflex by visual fixation and smooth pursuit. J Vestib Res 1994 Sep-Oct;4(5):347-53.

25. Herderman Susan J. Vestibular Rehabilitation. 2nd ed. Philadelphia, PA: F.A. Davis, 2000:391-2.

Sources

a. NeuroCom, International, Inc., Clackamas, OR

b. Life-Tech, Inc., Houston, TX

Vestibular Therapy and Ocular Dysfunction in Traumatic Brain Injury: A Case Study

David Malamut, M.A., P.T.

Introduction

The observations of vestibular therapists and the perspective of behavioral optometrists have generated promising and vital relationships among health care professionals. It is no novelty to the optometrist that issues related to vision might profoundly affect balance, gaze stability, fine and gross motor coordination, and cognitive function. Yet, in the nascence of vestibular therapy, visual function and visual rehabilitation were not frequently considered.

Years have passed since the closest thing to vestibular therapy was a battery of Cawthorne-Cooksey exercises.[1,2] Although these exercises, which were developed in the 1940s, acknowledge the connection between movement and vestibular recovery, the exercises were imprecise in their method of eliciting vestibulo-ocular function. New exercises have been developed, and various research studies suggest their efficacy.[3-5] Along with a more sophisticated understanding of the vestibulo-ocular reflex, there has developed an appreciation for the importance of normal extraocular function.[6-9] Treatment of the traumatic brain-injured (TBI) patient with vision therapy as well as vestibular exercise programs has become more commonplace.[10]

The case study that is later detailed in this chapter suggests the effectiveness of combining vestibular and visual intervention in improving overall vestibular function.

Neuroanatomy and Neurophysiology of the Vestibular System

The vestibular system is complex, involving interconnections among the inner ear, several portions of the brain, and specific muscles including those of the extraocular muscle and postural muscle systems. Included in the postural muscle system are the muscles of the back and lower extremities that keep the center of mass over the base of support. When sensory end organs in the inner ear receive information, it is relayed to the vestibular nuclei via the eighth cranial nerve. At the vestibular nuclei, the information is transformed into a message of action or inaction, and then sent to the appropriate neuromotor complexes (e.g., vestibulo-ocular reflex [VOR]

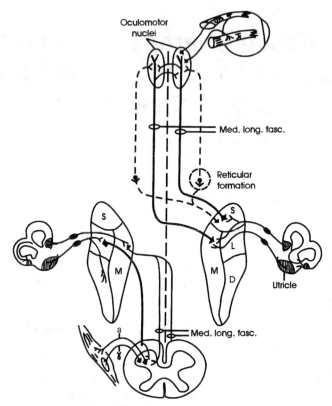

Figure 1. The vestibulo-ocular reflex arcs. S, L, M and D indicate the superior, lateral, medial and descending vestibular nuclei. The lateral vestibulospinal and medial vestibulospinal tracts are shown as heavy and light lines, respectively, beginning in the lateral vestibular nucleus. From Neurological Anatomy in Relation to Clinical Medicine, Third Edition by Alf Brodal. (New York: Oxford University Press, 1981) Used by permission of Oxford University Press, Inc.

and vestibulospinal reflex [VSR]). In addition, there is a proprioceptive feedback system that processes information related to the activity of these muscles and relays this information to the cerebellum. Error signals (e.g., retinal slip or inappropriate postural reactions) are recorded, analyzed, and adjusted for at the level of the cerebellum via pathways that connect to the aforementioned reflex arcs.[11]

Primary Function of the Vestibular Reflexes

The task of the vestibular system is to help maintain gaze stability when the head is moving quickly and to help maintain balance in that circumstance,[11] as well as in any in which information from other sources (visual and somatosensory) is lacking, confounding or inconsistent.

Balance and the vestibulospinal reflex

Balance is a multifactorial operation involving three dominant sensory functions: 1) somatosensory, 2) visual and 3) vestibular. It involves a combination of reflex and conscious activity that is impressive and too large a subject for this chapter. However, understanding the various sensory inputs that contribute to balance, as well as how they are integrated, is vital to grasping the importance of the vestibular system.

Under many circumstances, the information that we derive from our somatosensory and visual systems is adequate to the task of maintaining balance. When walking on a flat wooden, linoleum or cement floor, we obtain sufficient information from our feet (i.e., tactile) and joints (i.e., proprioceptive). In an environment that is devoid of moving objects, vision is an ideal contributor to steady balance. In fact, in these pristine circumstances, the somatosensory and visual systems are the rulers of balance, and the vestibular system is effectively irrelevant.

In reality, the above circumstances are unusual. Floors are often carpeted and imperfectly leveled. Outside terrain is typically irregular and of varying consistencies. Things are constantly moving in our visual fields. In short, somatosensory and visual reference points are not consistently reliable for maintenance of equilibrium. In these circumstances, a strong vestibular system is critical.[11] There exists a reliable and nonreferential source of balance information inside our ears. The inner ear houses not only the sensory end organ for hearing, but also the three semicircular canals and two otoliths that help us with gaze stability and balance.

Anatomy: Otoliths, gravity sensitivity and the vestibulospinal reflex

The otoliths (the utricle and the saccule) are the primary balance receptors of the inner ear. They provide information about the disposition of the head in relation to the gravitational axis and about the acceleration of the head in three dimensions.

Gravitational sensitivity is not a recent innovation in terms of evolution. It is precisely what allows for the ageotropic extension of vegetation. Mineral nutrients sink to the underside of stems and thereby increase growth, thus extending the vegetation away from the pull of gravity. In animals, this sensitivity has developed with greater precision and more impressive effect. As we move up the evolutionary scale, the fish demonstrate the greatest perfection of otolithic function. With the increased sophistication of the somatosensory and visual systems in mammals, the vestibular system devolved but remained pivotal among sensory sources of balance.

The otolith provides information through an ingenious arrangement of components that transform gravitational input into electrical energy. In the otolith, relatively heavy calcium carbonate crystals called otoconia sit on a gel matrix invaginated by hair cells. When shearing forces are exerted on these otoconia, the gel matrix is disturbed which, in turn, deflects the hair cells.[11]

Hair cells in the vestibular system are arranged in a "pipe organ" manner with smaller hair cells, the stereocilia, gathered in juxtaposition to a large hair cell, the kinocilium. In neutral circumstances, there is baseline firing of these cells. Deflection of stereocilia in the direction of the kinocilium excites the system, while deflection in the opposite direction inhibits the system.[12]

The utricle and saccule are somewhat boomerang-shaped and curved three-dimensionally. However, they each sit primarily in one plane. The utricle is for the most part in the horizontal plane, while the saccule is disposed sagittally.[12] The utricle and saccule, one each per ear, provide the nervous system with information related to linear acceleration of the head and disposition of the head in relation to gravity.

This extensive and detailed information is mapped on the otoliths, so that nervous system inputs result in the coordinated inhibition and excitation of postural muscles. The combination of sensory inputs and motor outputs under the regulatory influence of the cerebellum is the basis of the vestibulospinal reflex (VSR). In situations where the head is accelerating through space, rotating in any direction, or tilted, this reflex makes the adjustments necessary to maintain balance. When other sources of balance information are inadequate, confounding or conflicting, the vestibulospinal reflex mediates between the other sources. [1,13-15]

Semicircular canals and the vestibulo-ocular reflex

The semicircular canals provide information related to head rotation. They are arranged such that membranous curved pipes are housed inside identical bony semicircular structures with two different types of fluid, one between the two, the other within the membranous pipes. These two fluids are of different chemical compositions. The sensory transducer at the end of the pipe within the membrane is called the cupula. It has a "pipe organ" arrangement of hair cells within a gel substance[11] that is similar to that of the otolithic macula (i.e., the transducer of balance information).

When the head is rotated, the viscous endolymph on the inside of the membrane remains essentially still, while the membrane moves around it. In relation to the cupula, the relative movement of the fluid in the opposite direction causes deflection and a change in electrical energy.[16] As with the macula of the otolith, the direction of hair cell deflection will determine whether there is a decrease or increase in firing rate. As before, this information is mapped with effectors, which translate information into action. Each canal is coupled with a different set of extraocular muscles through the vestibulo-ocular reflex (VOR).[17]

Whenever we are able to keep our eyes fixated while our head is rotating at high speeds, we are using the VOR. At very slow speeds, our pursuit system suffices to stabilize the world by using the cervico-ocular reflex (COR). This reflex produces slow-phase eye movement via sensory inputs from the neck muscles and facet joints. During low frequency, brief head movement, the slow-phase eye movement that is produced is opposite in direction to that of the head.[18] Although the COR normally contributes approximately 15% of the compensatory eye movement, it can be trained in the absence of a VOR to stabilize gaze when the head moves in 20° oscillations at one Hz, as during VOR training sessions.[18] However, to move the head at two Hz or more and maintain stable fixation requires a strong VOR.

Functional aspects of the vestibular system
Visualize prehistoric man walking on the savannas of Africa engaged in his lifelong struggle to find prey and avoid predators. We could imagine no more vital reflex than that which allowed him to see and stay upright while mobile. Indeed, binocularity makes all the more compelling the capacity to turn the head with gaze and person stable. In man, the view of the surround depends on the mobility of the head. These faculties are no less vital in the modern world, which demands an analogous degree of acuity, mobility and polyattentiveness. Thus far, the description of these reflexes has not exhausted the role of the vestibular system in human function. It provides other inputs to gaze stability and balance, while contributing predictive postural adjustments and coordination in general.

Vestibular Dysfunctions
When there is a total absence of vestibular function, the substitution of information from other systems is required.[18,19] However, in most cases, an injury to, or pathology of, the vestibular system leaves a large portion of the system intact, as most disease involves unilateral lesions. In such cases, adaptation is possible.

Adaptation
Adaptation is the process by which the central nervous system corrects for a defective vestibular system. If a lesion at any location within the vestibular system has resulted in the processing of misinformation, the result is inappropriate effector activity. That activity may manifest itself on a sensory

level as blurred vision with head turning or as a sense of imbalance. The central nervous system has the capacity to correlate this misinformation with the extent of error in the response and reprogram the reflex through the cerebellum. More than half of the time our systems do this spontaneously without the intervention of the physical therapist.[6, 20] The vestibular therapist sees the unfortunate minority. There are some very particular reasons why these patients require vestibular therapy. To grasp these reasons, we must understand the meaning of adaptation.

Adaptation, in the context of this chapter, requires several components: 1) a discrete error signal, 2) an error signal of limited size (e.g., the target must be in focus) and 3) redundancy of error presentation.[11] The signal for vestibular adaptation is retinal slip (the movement of the image across the retina).[21] The major requirements of adaptation for the VOR are the following: 1) both eyes should provide the same error signal during a given speed of head movement; 2) the repeated movement of the head should not produce blurred or doubled vision, or the illusion of target movement (i.e., oscillopsia); and 3) the stimulation should last at least ninety seconds and be repeated every day, three times per day.

Symptoms/movement
Vestibular dysfunction not only causes reflex impairment, but also results in noxious symptoms including vertigo, lightheadedness, heavyheadedness, fullness in the ears, headache, nausea, fatigue, irritability, anxiety and cognitive impairment. All of these symptoms may be increased with vestibular stimulation, head movement and/or change in head position. Many patients avoid movement to decrease stimulation. However, without regular stimulation, the vestibular system is slow to adapt.

Spontaneous Recovery And Vestibular Rehabilitation
An important principle is that spontaneous recovery from vestibular insult is typical. Therefore, the therapist's role is that of vestibular detective. We can divide vestibular function into input and output. The input is the information (i.e., movement, positions of the body and/or head, and exposure to environments during daily activities or as part of a vestibular exercise program) that makes adaptation possible. The output is the body's translation of the input into the balance and gaze stability response. The appropriateness of the output is dependent upon adequacy of the vestibular apparatus with regard to the VSR function and the extraocular muscles with regard to the VOR function. The combination of input and output makes it possible for error signals to be read and corrected.

The Information: Frequency, Intensity, Duration, And Organization

The frequency, intensity, duration and organization of stimulating movement are major factors affecting the success of vestibular adaptation. Patients' fears inhibit them in the performance of symptom-provoking movements. Avoidance of these activities is a normal, but counterproductive, reaction. Without stimulation, there is no adaptation.

Typically, the patient who becomes dizzy from a particular activity (e.g., turning the head while walking) will curtail the activity or selectively avoid the specific portion of the movement that causes the symptoms. Similarly, a dizzy patient who is assigned a given exercise might refuse to perform that exercise or creatively, often subconsciously, alter the exercise to reduce its effects.

These habits die slowly. The therapist must increase the patient's willingness to move by establishing trust. Trust is possible if and only if the symptoms provoked are of tolerable intensity. Trust depends as much on the therapist's ability to convince the patient that regular symptom provocation is positive, as it does on the patient's absolute physical tolerance for this noxious experience. If the message is not convincingly conveyed to the patient, the amount of "tolerable" symptom provocation may not be enough to elicit adaptation. The vigilant and skilled therapist with requisite observational capability will notice and correct the subconscious alteration of exercise.

The monitoring of activities of daily living is important to the success of vestibular therapy. Type A personalities who work long, hard hours may bombard their vestibular systems to such a degree that they cannot perform the exercise or obtain any benefit from it. Patients with acquired brain injuries (ABI) are more problematic in that they not only overdose on daily activities, but often are unable to report what activities have and have not been done. ABI patients must be taught to monitor as well as moderate these activities to reap the benefits of therapy.

Effector Inadequacy

Another pitfall in the process of adaptation is the possible inadequacy of the effector organs of the reflex. The extraocular muscles are the prime movers of the VOR. Vestibular therapists direct patients to optometrists for a variety of reasons. For the purposes of this chapter, the discussion is limited to vergence, particularly convergence as related to vestibulo-ocular function.

207

Vergence Insufficiency and Maladaptation

Vergence is the disjunctive movement of the eyes that is required for precise ocular alignment to track objects moving in depth. Precise ocular alignment is needed to elicit binocular fusion and stereopsis.[22, 23] Since stereoscopic vision is required for accurate three-dimensional visual perception, it follows that appropriate vergence, too, is a prerequisite for accurate depth perception.

Vergence impairment has a profoundly negative effect upon vestibulo-ocular function. This is because in the absence of accurate vergence: 1) there is a disparity in the error signals (arising from the two eyes) going to the cerebellum, 2) the image is blurred or doubled, and therefore the error signal is too large, and 3) the error signal changes according to the angle of convergence and therefore is confusing and disorganized rather than redundant.

Prism Intervention

The literature suggests that where neuromotor control is the issue, vision therapy (VT) is the recommended treatment.[24-26] However, compensatory prisms are used when active VT is not feasible, or as a supplement to VT. It is important to note that a different type of adaptation from that discussed in reference to the vestibular system is at issue when discussing visual adaptation to prisms. Prism adaptation refers to the eyes' effectively nullifying the prismatic adjustment such that, over time, the prisms no longer compensate for the vergence insufficiency. Further, upon removal of the prisms, there can be an increase in the fusional impairment in proportion to the former prism correction. If the patient has normal neurological function, the effect of prism adaptation needs to be determined.[24] In contrast, patients with compromised neurological function (e.g., ABI secondary to trauma, stroke, tumor, aneurysm and postsurgical complications) frequently do not adapt to prisms. [9,27] The successful application of compensatory prism in this regard is illustrated in the following case study.

Case Study
Phase 1

GB was a 48-year-old white male construction worker who sustained a traumatic brain injury when he had a fall. GB was repairing a bridge connecting Manhattan and the Bronx on 9/14/94 when a four-ton piece of equipment broke loose from its moorings and struck him on the side of his head. He fell from the bridge and incurred further injury from collisions with portions of the bridge during his 20-foot descent into the river. He was pulled toward the river bottom by his 35-pound tool belt. GB was rescued by two co-workers who brought him, unconscious, to the surface. He remained unconscious for 20 minutes, until EMS workers arrived and administered oxygen.

GB was shuttled to an area hospital where he was treated for his wounds. Aided by his wife, GB left the hospital with no definitive diagnosis after being hospitalized for three days. Once he reached his home, continuous bleeding from his ear became evident. He was rushed to a second area hospital on 9/19/94. Superficial examination revealed a tender left shoulder with limited rotation, a large bruise in the upper right posterior thorax, blood in the upper right exterior auditory canal, and difficulty with right-sided hearing.

At GB's second visit (9/21/94) to this hospital, he complained of right-sided hearing impairment and manifested horizontal end-point nystagmus on right lateral gaze. GB was seen again on 10/11/94, by which time he could no longer hear through his right ear. Additional complaints were persistent left shoulder pain, limited movement of left shoulder due to pain, headaches and dizziness. The diagnosis was right temporal bone fracture with conductive hearing loss.

Surgery was performed on 12/12/94, at which time GB was found to have a suture line fracture in the posterior-superior portion of the length of the external auditory canal. The incus was dislocated, with the long process lateral to the chorda tympani. The stapes and malleus were normal. A Cartosh PORP was placed, which connected the stapes and malleus. The prosthesis fit well and allowed for appropriate movement of the stapes.

Three months after surgery, the audiogram revealed total recovery from his conductive right-sided hearing loss. GB complained of right temporomandibular joint pain radiating to the temporalis muscle, and he planned to see a dentist to address the problem. He continued to experience dizziness, which the doctor described as postconcussive.

Following continued vestibular complaints, a magnetic resonance imaging (MRI) scan was performed on 3/06/95. The findings were as follows: several punctate foci of high signal intensity were present within the white matter of the frontal lobes. These punctate foci were interpreted as being nonspecific and as representing areas of demyelination or gliosis. On 3/07/95, an electroencephalogram (EEG) was performed. The EEG results indicated bilateral cerebral dysfunction, which was manifested by excessive delta intensity. It was recommended that the EEG be repeated.

On 5/25/95, GB went for his six-month follow-up visit with the otolaryngologist who had performed the surgery in 1994. GB complained of right shooting preauricular pain radiating into the temporal region, hyperacusis (hypersensitivity to sound), and occasional episodes of dysequilibrium. The combination of symptoms and being unable to work had caused him to become depressed, for which he began receiving psychiatric treatment.

Several visits over the next year followed. On 10/15/96, the otolaryngologist who had performed the surgery examined GB and recommended vestibular therapy at the RUSK Institute of Rehabilitation Medicine.

On 11/05/96, another doctor examined GB. At this visit, he had a variety of complaints: headache around the right ear radiating to his right neck, constant imbalance and dizziness, decrease in hearing on the right, hyperacusis, constant tinnitus, temporomandibular joint discomfort, a foot spur, a lump sensation in his throat, retinal problems, and occasional blood circulation surges in his right ear. GB reported the use of a splint for his jaw and a cane for ambulation. He also relayed his surgeon's recommendation for vestibular rehabilitation. His medications included tranquilizers as well as pain relievers. The doctor performed an audiogram, electronystagmography, and brainstem evoked response test. The audiogram revealed a 9.4% impairment of hearing on the right side. Electronystagmography revealed a left unilateral weakness and a left-beating positional nystagmus. The brainstem evoked response test results were within normal limits bilaterally. Based upon these findings, this doctor also recommended vestibular therapy.

On 2/25/97, electromyography and a nerve conduction study were performed. The studies revealed a C5-6 radiculopathy, greater on the left than on the right, with denervation in paraspinal muscles. It was not until 4/09/97 that GB was evaluated at the RUSK Institute's Vestibular Unit.

Phase 2
Vestibular evaluation
Upon initial vestibular evaluation (4/09/97), GB complained of head pain, dizziness, vertical oscillopsia, a rocking sensation, and vertigo. He reported photosensitivity, dizziness with rapid head movement, hyperacusis, and an awareness of the sound of blood rushing in his right ear. Coordination tests demonstrated a slowing of movement with "finger to nose" testing as well as slowed, dysmetric movement with "finger to finger" and "past pointing" testing. Proprioception was impaired at the left great toe.

GB was able to stand in a sharpened Romberg position for 60 seconds with eyes open, but only 35 seconds with eyes closed. The results of the gaze stability exercise (i.e., turning the head side to side or up and down with a 30° magnitude while fixating a letter) were 8 horizontal head turns per minute and 12 vertical head turns per minute. However, during his performance of the gaze stability exercise, his vision became blurred, and he became dizzy. Appropriate adaptation when performing the gaze stability exercise requires the absence of blur, diplopia and oscillopsia.

GB was examined with Frenzel goggles. This device has high-powered convex lenses that markedly blur vision to prevent gaze fixation and magnify the patient's eyes to aid in the observation of eye movements. This revealed spontaneous nystagmus and head-shaking nystagmus with both vertical and horizontal head movements.

The driving force for most types of spontaneous nystagmus is the vestibular system. The imbalance of tonic signals arriving at the oculomotor neurons results in spontaneous nystagmus.

When there is an asymmetry of right versus left canal function, for example between right and left semicircular canals, post-headshaking nystagmus appears after less than 20 seconds of quick head shaking. This testing takes advantage of the fact that excitation of a canal is a more effective stimulus than inhibition, since an inhibited firing rate can not be driven below zero. Therefore, the velocity storage system (assuming that it is intact) will accumulate vestibular input such that the disparity between right and left canal function will result in slow eye movement toward the side of the lesion followed by a quick correction to the opposite side (horizontal post-headshaking nystagmus).

Both spontaneous and post-headshaking nystagmus, signs of vestibular dysfunction, are neurological in origin, unlike benign paroxysmal positional vertigo (BPPV) which is purely mechanical in origin. BPPV will be explained in greater detail in the next section.

Ambulation testing was performed using a cane over a 50-foot walking space. GB's habitual gait speed was 2.38 feet per second. When GB walked the same course while horizontally turning his head left and center every three steps, he walked at 0.56 feet per second. When he walked the same course while turning his head right and center every three steps, his gait speed was 1.06 feet per second. When GB walked the same course while continually turning his head horizontally from side to side and then vertically up and down, his gait speed was 0.96 and 0.93 feet per second, respectively. Age-related expected habitual gait is 4.11 feet per second. GB's Dizziness Handicap Inventory (DHI), a measure of the level of difficulty experienced as a result of dizziness or imbalance, was high with a score of 92 out of a possible 100.

The analog scale of the DHI allows a patient to estimate his level of symptomatology and functional impairment on a 100-point scale. GB's symptomatology score was 95 out of a possible 100, indicating an extremely high level of symptomatology. The analog scale relating to function requires the patient to estimate what percentage of normal his current performance is for a variety of functional activities. GB's rating was 92 out of 100, which indicated a very low level of function.

An Equitest (diagnostic testing using dynamic platform posturography) had been performed prior to our initial visit. The results revealed a severely abnormal composite score of 38% with a complete inability to employ the vestibular component of balance and deficits in the visual and, to a lesser extent, somatosensory components of balance.

Dynamic platform posturography is a "high tech" method of testing balance. It includes two major portions. The Sensory Organization Test (SOT) examines stability by quantifying sway, registered via pressure sensors in the platform. The platform is also sensitive to shear forces. Therefore the testee's use of the hip strategy, involving shear, as compared to ankle strategy, without shear, will correlate with sway, such that a picture of the appropriateness of strategies can be determined.

The second portion of the test, the Motor Control Test (MCT), includes portions which examine the latency of response to platform translation, amplitude scaling of responses, and adaptation of the patient to altered postural demands.

The portion of GB's Equitest to which we referred was the SOT. The composite score from this test gives a global sense of how stable the patient is by averaging the scores across all sensory conditions. GB's score was approximately half of the minimum score designated as normal.

The SOT presents six different conditions. Visual conditions change from eyes open in condition #1, to eyes closed in #2, to one hundred percent visual sway referencing in #3 (the background moves as much and in the same direction as the testee). In #4, #5, and #6, the visual conditions are repeated sequentially. During the first three conditions the platform is fixed; during the last three, the platform is one hundred percent sway referenced.

Since GB fell during each of three trials during condition #5, he received a score of zero, reflecting the absence of a vestibular component of balance. The vestibular component of balance is calculated by comparing norm adjusted scores from condition #5 to condition #1 where all sensory systems are available. The visual component is measured by comparing #4 to #1, while the somatosensory component is reflected in a comparison of #2 to #1.

Table 1. Exercises for Home Vestibular Therapy Regimen	
Purpose of Exercise	Exercise
Vestibuo-ocular	Gaze stability
Vestibulo-ocular substitute	Substitution for gaze stability, using imaginary targets with eyes closed
Vestibulo-ocular substitute	Substitution for gaze stability, with eyes open; move eyes, then move head
Ocular	Smooth pursuit
Balance	Romberg, with eyes open and eyes closed
Balance	Sit-to-stand, while fixating a target

Initial stage of vestibular therapy

Further assessment suggested that GB might have bilateral benign parox-ysmal positional vertigo (BPPV). This condition is characterized by epi-sodic vertigo with changes in head position in relation to the gravitational axis. It is a mechanical rather than neurological condition and may have been brought on by the head trauma of the accident. The blow to GB's head may have dislodged otoconia (calciferous granules) from the maculae of the utricles. These relatively heavy granules, when displaced, may have found their way to the semicircular canals. As a result of the change of head position in relation to the gravitational axis, these same crystals may move through the canal, pulled by gravity, and precipitate a flow of endolymph fluid inside the semicircular canals. This inappropriate flow may cause nystagmus via the pathway of the VOR. Episodic vertigo lasting several seconds, secondary to the dislodged, free-floating otoconia, is the result of this nystagmus. While nystagmus was not evident during the Hallpike-Dix testing, GB did complain of dizziness. Consequently we instructed him to perform the Brandt-Daroff habituation exercise, which can be used for both BPPV and nonspecified positional dizziness. At this time, GB also re-ported vertigo (duration: two to three hours) and lack of depth perception upon lateral head rotation. Based upon the results of the diagnostic testing, a home vestibular therapy regimen was designed using the exercises listed in Table 1.

GB was asked to perform the gaze stability exercise (bifixate on a station-ary target while turning one's head from side to side or up and down) while seated for one minute daily. Initially, all gaze stability exercises (including the substitution exercises to be described below) were performed using a tennis ball (i.e., a large target) rather than the ½- to ¾-inch letters that are typically used. Additionally, he was given a smooth pursuit exercise to im-prove visual tracking. Initially, GB manifested right-beating nystagmus and dizziness when performing the smooth pursuit. Sharpened Romberg with eyes open and ¾ sharpened Romberg with eyes closed, as well as sit-to-stand exercises in which GB moved from a seated to a standing position while viewing a target (to help reduce oscillopsia), were given to improve balance. Two substitution exercises were given to improve gaze stability with head movement: the first one is performed with the eyes closed, and the second one with the eyes open. Both of these substitution exercises are intended to substitute for an absent vestibulo-ocular reflex to maximize gaze stability with head movement.

The first substitution exercise utilizes imaginary targets and is similar to the gaze stability exercise except that it is performed with the eyes closed. GB was asked to look at a target letter in front of him, close his eyes, and imagine the target and its placement. Then GB rotated his head horizontally (or moved it up and down vertically), while moving his eyes to match the position of the imaginary target. GB was required to open his eyes at each extreme of movement to verify the accuracy of his eye movements in staying on the target of regard. If his eyes were off-target, then GB corrected the ocular alignment. The exercise was repeated for a given period of time, varying from one to five minutes. The second substitution exercise was one in which GB moved his eyes, and then his head, to aim towards one of two targets. This exercise is designed to help the patient develop a strategy for maintaining fixation on a target.

By the completion of the first two months of therapy, tracking had improved and the frequency of dizzy spells had decreased. At this time, turning was introduced, which induced nausea for GB. The magnitude of the turns was limited to ¼ turns. Head turning, either vertically or horizontally, was performed without ambulating through space. Convergence exercises were given to improve a significant vergence deficit.

One month later, GB was able to perform the substitution exercises while standing. Further, GB was able to perform a tandem walk with his hand on a wall for five to ten steps. By 8/11/97, GB was able to turn his head partially to the side, up or down and center every four steps while walking tentatively. GB was also able to walk tentatively on foam (one inch thick).

Until 7/24/98, GB was followed successively by two therapists, whose strategy it was to expose GB to both standard vestibular training and substitution exercises to improve function when adaptation was absent or slow. Convergence exercises were performed during the latter portion of this period.

Table 2.
GB's Subjective Ratings at Varying Stages of the Vestibular Therapy Regimen.

Scale	Initial Physical Therapy Evaluation	Pre-Optometric Evaluation	Post-Optometric Evaluation
Dizziness Handicap Inventory	92	Not assessed	66
Analog Scale: Symptoms	95	94	42
Analog Scale: Function	96	89	39
Functional Checklist: Selected Areas of Function			
Transportation	0	10	40
Shopping	0	10	40
Indoor walking	5	10	50
Outdoor walking	0	10	60
Walking in darkness	0	5	30
Household activities	0	0	20
Self care	0	20	80
Work	0	0	20
Recreation	0	5	20
Social activities	0	10	20
Cognitive activities	0	5	20

The three scales used were the Dizziness Handicap Inventory (DHI) scale, analog scale (for symptoms and level of function), and functional checklist. For the DHI and the analog scale, the rating is from 0 to 100. Zero represents no difficulty with dizziness, no symptoms, and maximum function, while 100 represents the maximum amount of difficulty with dizziness, the maximum severity of symptoms, and minimal function. For the functional checklist, the patient assigns a percent value between 0 and 100 as a measure of the percentage of normal that the patient performs in select areas of function. For the functional checklist, 0 represents as far from normal as possible, and 100 represents normal.

By the end of this period the oscillopsia had diminished, and balance without head movement was somewhat improved. Gaze stability with head movement remained poor. GB continued to perform the gaze stability exercise at seven head rotations per minute. In contrast, the expected age-related performance is 120 head rotations per minute. A substitution exercise, where GB turned his shoulders while maintaining ocular and head fixation on a stationary target, was impossible. Although GB's symptomatology had lessened as long as his head was stationary, he still had no gaze stability with head movement and, furthermore, was unable to turn his head while walking with a steady gaze and equilibrium. GB remained unstable in any situation requiring sensory integration. His subjective evaluations (self-evaluation) showed small improvements on the analog scale. Although changes in symptomatology were small, his function did improve moderately for most activities, according to the analog scale (see Table 2).

Phase 3

On 7/24/98, GB switched vestibular therapists for the final time. Two major issues were revisited: gaze stability and vergence. The speed of the gaze stability exercise had not increased in over one year. Vergence training was revisited, but the nearpoint of convergence went only from 24 inches to 22 inches over a two-week period. GB was still unable to walk and turn his head without gaze instability and saccadic movement of the eyes. Head movement while walking was attempted via the eye/head movements used to perform the "two target" exercise. GB was asked to face one target, then, without turning his head, to look at a second target. Then GB was asked to turn his head to catch up with his eyes. This task was repeated and then attempted while walking. GB's eye/head movements became slightly more fluid, but remained slow.

On 10/21/98, GB underwent an ocular and visual evaluation by an optometrist from the Head Trauma Vision Rehabilitation Unit of the State University of New York, State College of Optometry. For the purpose of this chapter, the most important diagnosis was intermittent alternating exotropia at distance and near. A program of optometric vision therapy was not feasible at that time because of financial and other constraints. Consequently, compensatory (fusional) prisms (a total of four prism diopters base-in) were prescribed. The optometrist and physical therapist discussed the findings, and the physical therapist monitored GB's program to coordinate therapy with progressive prism use, as recommended by the optometrist. The plan was to monitor the effect of the prisms in terms of symptomatology and effect on the vestibular rehabilitation program. GB was instructed to increase his time wearing the prism spectacles gradually. By 12/02/98, GB was able to wear the glasses for three consecutive hours daily. When wearing the prism, he was able to fuse a target at a distance of one foot. Further, GB's speed of performing the gaze stability exercise increased by fourfold with steady fixation. His ability to perform the substitution exercise of fixating a letter while rotating his trunk also improved. By the end of December 1998, GB reported increased confidence walking outdoors, walking up steps without holding rails, and increased depth perception.

By 4/28/99, GB progressed to performing the gaze stability exercise with approximately 70 head rotations per minute while wearing the prismatic spectacle correction. Further, when wearing the prisms, GB was able to walk backwards, walk on a treadmill (without holding on) for four minutes at 1.0 mile per hour, and move his head quickly from side to side while walking.

As of 8/11/99, GB could perform the gaze stability exercise while walking and holding a target in his hands. His habitual gait speed had improved to 3.85 feet per second. Within one month, he was able to walk while turning his head (from side to side, up and down, and diagonally) with every step, stand on five inches of foam with his eyes closed while maintaining his balance, and walk backwards without loss of balance. By mid-October 1999 GB was able to perform the horizontal gaze stability exercise at over 80 head rotations per minute and the vertical gaze stability at 100 head rotations per minute. Further, he now walked unaided and carried his cane only as a precaution.

The success of incorporating fusional prisms with GB's vestibular therapy was not confined to gaze stability. With the improvement in his convergence, the visual system became an effective input to the balance system. In addition, improved dynamic visual acuity due to use of the VOR freed the patient to turn his head without creating a confusing visual surround. The patient began to stimulate the VSR with head movement and improved vestibularly-mediated balance function. He was able to stand on 5 inches of foam with feet together for 90 seconds, when previously he had been unable to stand with feet apart on 2 inches of foam. Without input from the eyes (i.e., eyes closed scenario) and with confusing input from the feet or somatosensory system (i.e., foam or compliant surface), the only sensory input for balance is the inner ear (i.e., the vestibular system). Therefore, improvement under these circumstances is indicative of vestibular adaptation in the absence of somatosensory and visual stimulation contribution.

Over the course of treatment, GB's score on the Dizziness Handicap Inventory scale improved from 92 (pre-optometric intervention) to 66 (post-optometric intervention with subsequent vestibular rehabilitation). Analog scale measurements improved by more than half relative to the results obtained prior to the optometric evaluation. Functional checklist findings showed 400 percent improvement or greater in all but social activities (see Table 2).

Summary
As in GB's case, the enhancement of two of the three sensory functions contributing to balance (visual and vestibular) will heighten the capacity of the patient to integrate sensory information. Conversely, if the patient inappropriately ignores or attends to visual information because it is confusing, the integration process is confounded, and balance is compromised.

This discussion has been extended to raise additional issues which improved convergence brings to the balance table: 1) enhanced visually-mediated balance function, 2) improved vestibulospinal reflex facilitated by the improvement of vestibulo-ocular reflex resulting in a willingness to turn one's head and 3) improved sensory integration. With continued observation of GB and others with similar convergence deficits, more information will be gathered regarding the above. What is clear, however, is the dramatic improvement in dynamic gaze stability, and the fact that the gains achieved through the use of fusional prisms were subsequently transferred to situations in which they were not used. Thus, GB's nearpoint of convergence without the prism glasses improved to 15 inches, whereas previously it had been beyond 3 feet.

The striking progress of the patient in gaze stability with head movement after a long period of potential recovery quite strongly suggests that the pivotal event was the introduction of prisms. Two additional points must be made in this regard. First, while optometric vision therapy might have been a viable option, the patient was unable to obtain insurance coverage for this treatment. Second, had an earlier optometric evaluation been possible, there is the distinct possibility that GB's rehabilitative progress might have been significantly enhanced. Ideally, this case study will not only encourage but also expand further research on the subject to include investigating the following three aspects of balance function which we feel are influenced by improved convergence: 1) visually-mediated balance, 2) vestibulospinal reflex function and 3) sensory integration.

References

1. Black FO, Nashner L. Vestibulo-spinal control differs in patients with reduced and distorted vestibular function. Acta Otolaryngol Suppl 1984; 406:110-4.

2. Cooksey FS. Rehabilitation in vestibular injuries. Proc Royal Soc Med 1946; 39:273.

3. Herdman SJ. Exercise strategies for vestibular disorders. Ear Nose Throat J 1989; 68(12):961-4.

4. Herdman SJ. Assessment and treatment of balance disorders in the vestibular-deficient patient. In: Duncan P, ed. Balance Proceedings of the APTA Forum. Nashville: American Physical Therapy Association, 1990: 87.

5. Norre ME. Treatment of unilateral vestibular hypofunction. In: Oosterveld WJ, ed. Otoneurology. New York: John Wiley, 1984: 23.

6. Pfaltz CR. Vestibular compensation: physiological and clinical aspects. Acta Otolaryngol 1983; 95:402-6.

7. Collewijn H, Martins AJ, Steinman RM. Compensatory eye movements during active and passive head movements: fast adaptation to changes in visual magnification. J Physiol 1983; 340:259-86.

8. Lisberger SG, Miles FA, Optican LM. Frequency-selective adaptation: evidence for channels in the vestibulo-ocular reflex. J Neurosci 1983;3(6):1234-44.

9. Godaux E, Halleux J, Gobert C. Adaptative change of the vestibulo-ocular reflex in the cat: the effects of a long-term frequency-selective procedure. Exp Brain Res 1983;49(1): 28-34.

10. Ciuffreda KJ, Suchoff IB, Marrone MA, Ahmann EB. Oculomotor rehabilitation in the traumatic brain-injured patient. J Behav Optom 1996;7(2):31-8.

11. Herdman SJ. Vestibular Rehabilitation. Philadelphia: F.A. Davis, 1994:3-31.

12. Furman J, Cass FP. Balance Disorders: A Case Study Approach. Philadelphia: F.A. Davis, 1994:4-15.

13. Nashner L, Black FO, Wall C III. Adaptation to altered support and visual conditions during stance: patients with vestibular deficits. J Neurosci 1982;2(5):536-44.

14. Black FO et al. Abnormal postural control associated with peripheral vestibular disorders. In: Pompeiano O, Allum JHJ, eds. Vestibular Control of Posture and Locomotion. Progress in Brain Research, Vol 76. Amsterdam: Elsevier, 1988: 263.

15. Shumway-Cook A, Horak FB. Assessing the influence of the sensory interaction on balance. Phys Ther 1986; 66(10):1548-50.

16. Wilson VJ, Jones MJ. Mammalian Vestibular Physiology. New York: Plenum Press, 1979.

17. Baloh RW, Honnrubia V. Clinical Neurophysiology of the Vestibular System. Philadelphia: F.A. Davis, 1990:52.

18. Bronstein AM, Hood JD. The cervico-ocular reflex in normal subjects and patients with absent vestibular function. Brain Res 1986; 373(1-2):399-408.

19. Kosai T, Zee DS. Eye-head coordination in labyrinthine-defective human being. Brain Res 1978; 144(1):123-41.

20. Igarashi M. Vestibular compensation: an overview. Acta Otolaryngol Suppl 1984; 406:78-82.

21. Miles FA, Eighmy BB. Long-term adaptive changes in primate vestibulo-ocular reflex: I. Behavioral observations. J Neurophys 1980; 43(5):1406-25.

22. Leigh, Zee D. The Neurology of Eye Movements, 2nd ed. Philadelphia: F.A. Davis, 1991:264-5.

23. Ciuffreda KJ, Tannen B. Eye Movement Basics for the Clinician. St. Louis: Mosby Year Book, 1995.

24. North R, Henson DB. Adaptation to prism-induced heterophoria in subjects with binocular vision or asthenopia. Am J Optom Physiol Opt 1981;58(9):746-52.

25. Schor C. Influence of accommodative and vergence adaptation on binocular motor disorders. Am J Optom Physiol Opt 1988; 65(6): 464-75.

26. Milder DG, Reinecke RD. Phoria adaptation to prisms. Arch Neurol 1983; 40(6):339-42.

27. Welch RB, Goldstein G. Prism adaptation and brain damage. Neuropsychologia 1972; 10:387-94.

Vestibular Dysfunction Associated with Traumatic Brain Injury: Collaborative Optometry and Physical Therapy Treatment

Lynn Fishman Hellerstein, O.D.
Patricia A. Winkler, M.S., P.T., NCS

Introduction

Sensory inputs from the vestibular, visual and somatosensory systems are integrated for orientation to the environment and for balance.[1,2] When a patient sustains a traumatic brain injury, one or more of the three systems may be injured. As a result of the injury a lack of, or conflict in, sensory messages results in symptoms including vertigo, dizziness, poor balance, moving or unstable visual world, and a variety of others. Treatment often includes vestibular therapy and optometric rehabilitative vision therapy.

This chapter reviews the neuroanatomy and neurophysiology of the vestibular system. In addition, an in-depth case study is presented to demonstrate our collaborative approach in treating this type of patient based on the neurophysiologic symptoms presented.

Background Information
Neuroanatomy and neurophysiology of the vestibular system [3,4]

The vestibular system includes the peripheral vestibular receptors in the inner ear. The vestibular pathways including the vestibular nerve, the brainstem vestibular nuclei and the older parts of the cerebellum (vestibulocerebellum).

Peripheral receptors

Peripheral receptors in the inner ear, or labyrinths, consist of three semicircular canals, which are oriented at 90° with respect to each other (horizontal or lateral, anterior or superior, and posterior) and the otoliths (utricle and saccule). Each canal is filled with fluid (endolymph), which responds to fast head motions. The canals have a widening at their base (ampulla). The cupula is a gelatinous plug that extends from the bottom to the top of the ampulla and contains the hair or nerve cells that conduct the neurological impulses from the inner ear to the brain via the vestibular nerve.

Movement of the head bends the cupula and hair cells, which depolarizes the vestibular nerve. At rest, the firing rate of the vestibular nerves is about 90 spikes/second. Turning of the head causes increased firing ipsilateral to the movement and decreased firing in the corresponding canal on the contralateral side by an equal amount. This is called a push-pull system.

The two otolith organs, the utricle and saccule, also contain hair cells. These hair cells project into a gelatinous membrane and are covered with otoconia to add weight. The added weight allows them to bend with gravity, thus sensing head tilt. They also respond to linear acceleration in the horizontal and vertical planes.

The vestibular pathways and oculomotor pathways

Most canal and otolith nerve fibers go to the vestibular nuclei in the brainstem via the vestibular nerve. These nuclei process vestibular, visual, somatosensory and auditory information. Efferent fibers proceed from the vestibular nuclei to the oculomotor nuclei for control of the vestibulo-ocular reflex (VOR). Other efferent fibers proceed from the vestibular nuclei to the spinal cord for motor control of balance through the vestibulospinal reflex (VSR).

Many fibers from the vestibular nuclei proceed directly to the cerebellum. The cerebellum controls and modifies the VOR as well as adjusting the gain for saccadic eye movements, vergence movements and balance reflexes. Information from the visual cortex is also transmitted to the cerebellum. This information then proceeds to the vestibular nuclei and to the oculomotor muscles for control of the optokinetic nystagmus (OKN) reflexes (which stabilize vision during sustained rotation), as well as optokinetic after nystagmus (OKAN), which prevents vertigo after rotation has ceased. Information from the vestibular nuclei also projects to the reticular formation which has vomiting centers, attention and alertness centers, and efferent projections to the spinal cord for balance reflexes and to the oculomotor system for eye movements.

Functional aspects of the three systems

Sensory inputs from the vestibular, visual and somatosensory systems are integrated for orientation to the environment and for balance. This information is integrated and results in normal balance responses and spatial orientation. Each of these sensory systems has specific tasks and deficiencies.[1, 2]

The vestibular system
The vestibular system has three main functions:

1. provides posture and balance control via the vestibulospinal tract (VSR). This includes orientation to gravity through the otoliths;

2. provides a mechanism to distinguish movement in the environment from self motion;

3. maintains visual fixation during head and/or body movement via the VOR.

The vestibular system alone is unable to distinguish body tilt or body motion from head motion.

The somatosensory system
The somatosensory system (information from muscle and joint receptors) provides information on the relationship of one body segment to another and of the feet to the support surface. This system also provides the first line of adjustment for regaining balance during perturbations. The somatosensory system alone is unable to distinguish surface tilts from head tilts.

The visual system
The visual system provides vertical orientation, detects optic array movement and provides depth perception of objects moving towards/away from the individual. The visual system alone is inadequate in distinguishing movement of the environment from movement of the body.

Sensory integration and sensory conflict
People may use any combination of senses to maintain equilibrium, depending on the environmental conditions. All three senses described above are used in most situations to correct and provide balance responses. When sensory information from one of these three senses disagrees with that of another, a sensory conflict is said to occur. An example is standing while a large ball rolls toward you. As the ball moves toward you, the retinal image movement is the same as if you were to lean forward toward the ball and the ball were still. The brain resolves the problem of whether you leaned forward or the ball moved forward by assessing information from the somatosensory system to determine if the ankle rotated and the calf muscles elongated. The brain also assesses vestibular system output to determine if fluid moved in the semicircular canals or whether the otoliths detected forward or translatory movement.

In general, a sensory conflict is resolved by utilizing the sensory system whose information matches that information provided by the vestibular system. Thus, the vestibular sense is used as an internal reference to determine the accuracy of the other two senses. Sensory conflicts result in dizziness unless resolved rapidly. Patients with vestibular dysfunction use vision as their primary orientation system,[5] even if vision is impaired and thus results in even greater sensory conflict.

Symptoms of vestibular dysfunction [6-8]

Vertigo is the hallmark symptom of acute vestibular lesions. Vertigo may be an illusion of motion, usually a sense of rotation of self or the world if from the semicircular canals, whereas the otoliths provide a sense of rocking or of linear displacement (falling or floating). Vertigo results from unequal firing between the two opposite vestibular nerves or damage in the vestibular nuclei.

Dizziness results from a disruption in sensory integration. Less specific than vertigo, symptoms include lightheadedness, "swimmy," giddy, fuzzy, foggy, spaciness, blurred vision, motion sickness, sense of imbalance, disoriented, intoxicated, etc. Patients may use many descriptors. The origin may be due to vestibular, somatosensory and/or visual dysfunctions. Dizziness may also be cardiac, metabolic, psychological or medication related.

Gaze instability results from a disruption of the VOR. Patients may describe their visual world as jumping, bouncing, jerking or moving with them (oscillopsia). They may complain of object movement when turning their head or deterioration of visual acuity during or immediately after rapid head motion.

Postural instability results from disruption in the VSR. Patients may lack certain balance motor strategies or may use the wrong strategy for the conditions of the environment. They may also have imbalance secondary to a lack of orientation to the environment.

Nystagmus is an involuntary, rhythmic oscillation of the eyes that is typically conjugate. Pathological nystagmus includes:

1) Spontaneous nystagmus results from tonic imbalance in the vestibular nuclei. Spontaneous nystagmus occurs after acute lesions and usually lasts 24 hours. Nystagmus from the peripheral vestibular system is easily inhibited with visual fixation. Spontaneous nystagmus may also occur after central lesions of the brainstem or cerebellum. It is not easily inhibited with visual fixation.

2) Positional nystagmus is induced by a change in static head position. There are three types of positional nystagmus, each with different pathologies:

a) paroxysmal nystagmus occurs with stimulation of the canals, lasts seconds, then is gone;

b) central nystagmus occurs with damage to the central vestibular system, and lasts minutes or longer;

c) static nystagmus occurs with a change of head position in relation to gravity. It continues at the same frequency as long as the specific position is maintained. It can be suppressed with visual fixation, and it occurs with lesions to the otolith system.

3) Gaze-evoked nystagmus occurs when patients shift their gaze from the primary position. It is usually of central origin and is common in patients with multiple sclerosis, brain injury and congenital lesions.

Visual system problems[9-13] include dysfunctions of accommodation, vergence, version, visual perceptual deficits and visual field loss. OKN and OKAN can be abnormal as well. It is noteworthy that some patients report that visual stimulation produces nausea, vomiting and sweating. This is probably the result of flawed intersensory matching of information sent by the vestibular and visual systems at the nausea (vomiting) centers of the reticular formation.

Evaluation of the patient with vestibular dysfunction

A thorough history can begin to identify which of the three sensory systems may be causing the dizziness and imbalance symptoms. If a patient has symptomatology when performing tasks such as making the bed, walking up and down stairs, reaching or looking up, riding in a car around curves, riding elevators, making quick stops, etc., then symptoms are most likely directly related to vestibular stimulation. Dizziness or imbalance occurring only with unusual head or body positions such as rolling over and sitting up in bed may be a hypersensitivity to stimulation of the vestibular canals in general or a single canal problem (benign positional vertigo).

Visual dependency and hypersensitivity may be the primary problem if visual stimulation alone is causing imbalance and dizziness. These symptoms are reported occurring most often when a patient is shopping in crowded stores, grocery shopping, or in visually busy environments, such as rows of trees along the road. This problem is the visual equivalent of vestibular hypersensitivity. The patient is unable to habituate or ignore the movements in the visual surround.

Inadequate use of somatosensory cues may be apparent in a patient who has difficulty walking in the dark, falling, or losing balance when closing their eyes. Sensory selection may be a problem when the patient's dizziness is provoked while in a land or water vehicle or when positioned on a moving surface. In these cases, one of the three systems signals lack of movement (i.e., the somatosensory system), while the others signal that movement is really occurring. If the patient selects the somatosensory system as being the "correct" reading, then dizziness may result.

A patient with signs and symptoms suggesting a vestibular dysfunction requires a full medical workup. Often a neurologist and/or otologist has evaluated the patient and ordered appropriate medical tests including magnetic resonance imaging (MRI), electronystagmogram (ENG), hearing test, pressure tests for Meniere's disease and testing for fistulas. Referral to a neurologic physical therapist with vestibular treatment experience and to an optometrist with rehabilitation/vision therapy experience is appropriate for evaluation and treatment. To illustrate the collaborative evaluation and treatment process, a case study is presented.

Case Study
History
BP is a 31-year-old female who was involved in a motor vehicle accident (MVA) that occurred 6/21/91. Her seat belt restrained her, and she had to be cut from the car. She was unconscious for a few minutes at the scene of the accident. Direct trauma occurred to the head and neck as well as both knees. There was a right brachial plexus injury. Other symptoms included dizziness, nausea, blurred vision and imbalance. On 10/18/95, she was hit from behind in a second MVA, sustaining whiplash and experiencing increased dizziness and nausea.

There was no previous history of trauma to the head, neck or back, and no pertinent family medical history for diabetes, glaucoma, cataracts, hypertension, strabismus or retinal problems was noted. There was a positive family history for arthritis.

Visual history
Her last vision evaluation was 1986. No glasses or other interventions were recommended.

Neuropsychological testing
Documented problems included memory loss, attention/concentration problems, poor recall of newly acquired information, slowed information processing, word finding difficulties, poor reading comprehension, and difficulty with writing. A nonverbal learning deficit was diagnosed.

Medications
Isocet for headache, Amitriptyline, birth control pills, and Tagamet for ulcers.

Occupation

Homemaker. BP was a volunteer for the Brain Injury Foundation.

BP's neurologist diagnosed traumatic brain injury and vestibular dysfunction on 9/28/94.

Treatment included physical therapy for neck pain, TMJ dysfunction, knee problems and gait dysfunction. An occupational therapist had seen her for perceptual problems and for assistance performing activities of daily living (ADL). A speech-language pathologist treated BP for cognitive problems. Auditory biofeedback was given for stress reduction. BP was restricted from sports and certain motor activities such as tennis, biking, riding and weight lifting.

Subjective reports

BP reported frequent headaches, dizziness, nausea, blurred vision and difficulty reading. It was evident that her frequent loss of place adversely affected reading and comprehension. Dizziness occurred when shopping, walking in the dark, driving a car, and in moving and/or highly stimulating visual environments. The level of dizziness was reported as averaging an eight out of ten when walking (ten being so dizzy that one cannot stand up and zero being a total lack of dizziness). BP experienced dizziness when standing or sitting with her eyes closed, but not when lying down except with very rapid head motions.

Optometric evaluation

BP was evaluated four years after her injury. No medical provider had recommended a vision evaluation during her treatment following the accident.

The external examination was unremarkable for both eye and adnexa. Pupils were equal, round and responded to light; no Marcus Gunn response was apparent. Slit lamp biomicroscopy was unremarkable for both eyes. Intraocular pressures were 15 mm Hg OU by applanation tonometry.

The dilated fundus examination revealed cup to disc ratios (C/D) 0.1 OD, 0.1 OS, normal macular and foveal areas, intact vascular trees OU, and no pathology in the retinal periphery.

Initial testing revealed esophoria at distance and near, receded nearpoint of convergence, reduced fusion ranges, alternating suppression, decreased stereopsis, reduced positive relative accommodation, mildly reduced visual acuity at distance and near, and mild hyperopia with astigmatism. Pursuits and saccades were full, but with frequent loss of the target. BP demonstrated tearing, discomfort and difficulty integrating pursuit with cognitive tasks. Visual spatial/localization testing was variable and inconsistent. Visual fields revealed a normal blind spot; however, there was peripheral decrease in sensitivity not consistent with specific neurologic pattern. The visual fields may reflect a disturbance in attentional mechanisms revealed when executing dual tasks.[9] Table 1 provides more specific information.

Table 1. Optometric Findings		
Test	Pre-Treatment 8/10/95	Post-Treatment 6/12/96
Visual acuity (unaided) Distance Near	20/25 monocular 20/30 monocular	20/25 monocular 20/30 monocular
Distance refraction	OD +1.00-.50X25 (20/25) OS +1.00-.50X165 (20/25)	OD +1.25-.50X25 (20/20) OS +1.25-.50X165 (20/20)
Visual fields	Normal blind spot. Peripheral decrease in sensitivity not consistent with specific neurologic pattern.	Normal visual field
Cover test distance	2-3$^\Delta$ esophoria	orthophoria
Cover test near	6$^\Delta$ esophoria	4$^\Delta$ esophoria
Nearpoint of convergence	4/6 inches, discomfort and blur reported	½ inch, no discomfort
Phoria in phoropter (horizontal): Distance Near; plano lens Near; subjective lens Near; +1.00D add over subjective Phoria in phoropter (vertical)	3$^\Delta$ 9$^\Delta$ 3$^\Delta$ orthophoria orthophoria	orthophoria 8$^\Delta$ esophoria 3$^\Delta$ esophoria 2$^\Delta$ exophoria orthophoria
Vergences: Distance base out Distance base in Near base out Near base in	12/6$^\Delta$ 6/0$^\Delta$ 12/6$^\Delta$ 12/6$^\Delta$	20/10$^\Delta$ 9/4$^\Delta$ 18/14$^\Delta$ 20/16$^\Delta$
Accommodative status: PRA NRA Crossed cylinder Near retinoscopy	1.50D 3.25D +2.00D lag over subjective +2.25D lag over habitual (no Rx)	2.50D 3.25D +2.00D lag over subjective + 1.00D over Rx
Stereopsis	Randot 70 sec arc	Randot 20 sec arc
Cheiroscopic tracing, Van Orden Star	Alternating suppression with disorganized pattern	Stable pattern, no suppression
Ocular motilities	Pursuit and saccades: concomitant with full excursions in all fields of gaze, but with frequent loss of the target. Tearing, discomfort and difficulty integrating pursuit with cognitive tasks.	Ocular motilities: Full and unrestricted, no discomfort or nausea
Visual spatial/localization	Visual midline and localization (pointing to a ball with arms length) were variable and inconsistent	Visual midline and localization were stable and normal

227

Physical therapy examination

BP's neurologist referred her four years after the injury in 1995 for vestibular physical therapy.

Cerebellar testing revealed difficulty on the finger-to-nose test with the left hand. The heel-up-to-shin test showed ataxic movements bilaterally. No movement or resting tremors were noted. Balance, gait and oculomotor functions were all abnormal. Strength and lower extremity flexibility were within functional limits of normal. Hallpike testing (a test in supine position with head extended and rotated) for benign positional vertigo was negative.

Physical therapist's assessment: BP was visually dominated for her balance reactions, and visual motion caused dizziness and nausea. She had head motion provoked imbalance, nausea and dizziness. There was minimal use of somatosensory cues for balance reactions. Table 2 provides more detailed information.

Table 2. Physical Therapy Findings		
Test	Pre-Treatment 10/10/95	Post-Treatment 2/26/96
Dizziness Borg scale of 0=no dizziness, 10=so dizzy you would fall down	Constant dizziness in sitting or standing position when eyes are closed. Level 8, when in the dark, when in grocery stores, in environments with much movement (malls, etc.) and with head motion in walking or standing. Also with eye tracking activities	No dizziness with eyes closed. Level 0 except for level 1 or 2 when backing up in the car.
Nausea Borg scale: 0=none, 10=vomiting	Level 8 with activities as listed under dizziness above	None
Oculomotor function	VOR—blurring and object movement with head motion above 1 Hz Corrective saccades with smooth pursuit	Normal VOR Normal smooth pursuit
Balance Tested with feet together	Eyes open=WNL Eyes closed=falls backward immediately Head turning=falls in 5 seconds	All 30 seconds without symptoms or increased sway
Balance Tested standing on foam	Eyes open=increased sway Eyes closed=falls backward immediately Head turning=unable	All 30 seconds and without symptoms or increased sway
Single leg standing	20 seconds	30 seconds
Motor strategies	Poor hip strategy Ankle strategy was WNL	All motor strategies WNL
Gait	No head or trunk movement with walking. Multiple step-outs with head turning and after turning around 180°	Normal head motion and trunk rotation. No losses of balance or step-outs with head motion.

Diagnoses

The collaborative diagnoses from the otologist, neurologist, physical therapist and optometrist were:

1. traumatic brain injury with central vestibular dysfunction (injury to the brainstem and/or cerebellum);

2. convergence excess, accommodative dysfunction, oculomotor dysfunction, uncorrected low hyperopia with astigmatism, visual-spatial deficits, abnormal visual field;

3. loss of ability to use somatosensory input for balance responses with substitution of visual system to enhance balance; and disruption of balance from vestibular stimulation (head movement).

Rehabilitative management

At the time of initiating therapy for her dizziness, imbalance and visual problems, BP was no longer in treatment with other health care providers except her primary physician, a neurologist. BP had discontinued all other therapies. A combination of vestibular physical therapy (PT) and rehabilitative vision therapy (VT) was prescribed. It is important to note that PT and VT were initiated four years after the initial injury. Therefore, spontaneous recovery was not logically a factor. The delay in referral for PT and VT was due to the lack of knowledge of medical providers in understanding and utilizing such therapy options. BP had a total of seven treatments in PT and twenty treatments in VT concurrent with home therapy procedures.

Vision management

Vision management included distance glasses: OD +1.00-.50 X 25, OS +1.00-.50 X 165. While the distance prescription did not initially enhance visual acuity, BP reported improvement in ocular comfort. A near Rx of OD +1.75-.50 X 25, OS +1.75-.50 X 165 was also prescribed. Bifocals were not recommended because of the patient's symptoms of dizziness and visual overstimulation.[14]

Rehabilitative VT was initiated weekly with home therapy techniques to be completed daily. The treatment progressed from equalizing monocular skills to improving binocular skills. Vision therapy techniques, as listed in Table 3, were employed to improve oculomotor, accommodative, vergence, spatial awareness/localization, visual information processing and visual motor skills. Vision therapy proceeded slowly, as BP could not tolerate quick visual movement or changes. As visual skills improved, techniques to include body movement and balance were added. Adaptive strategies to decrease the symptoms of dizziness and nausea included use

Table 3. Vision Therapy Techniques*	
Oculomotor techniques	1. Eye "calisthenics" 2. Thumb pursuits 3. Marsden ball techniques 4. Pursuits and saccades while standing on balance board, progressing to eyes stationary while moving head, head tilt while performing pursuits and saccades 5. Pursuits and saccades while walking, running
Alignment & vergence	1. Brock string 2. Vectograms 3. Aperture rule 4. Prism rock
Visual information processing	1. Parquetry block series 2. Visualization strategies
Accommodative techniques	1. +/- lens flippers 2. Hart chart 3. Mental minus
Spatial awareness	1. Kirschner arrow charts 2. SUNY Visual Motor Series 3. Yoked prisms with body movement 4. Cross crawls
Visual motor techniques	1. Marsden ball hitting on balance board 2. Peg rotator 3. Trampoline fixations 4. Pitch back activities

*Virtually all of these techniques are described in various chapters in Press LJ, ed. Applied Concepts in Vision Therapy. St. Louis: Mosby 1997.

of peppermint candy, spotting techniques to suppress VOR subsequent to head/body rotations, and utilization of proprioceptive information (i.e., wall pushups, joint compression [pressing on head or shoulders], pushing or carrying weighted objects).

Physical therapy management

The physical therapist addressed the dizziness with strategies to decrease the conflicting information on position and movement. Because BP was using her visual system as her main input for balance (even with the visual dysfunctions documented earlier), she was very unstable in dynamic environments. Primarily, she was unable to distinguish environmental movement from self movement. Initial treatment stressed use of somatosensory inputs from the skin, muscles and joints while vision was occluded. These activities were begun in sitting and standing positions. The initial program emphasized feeling still and not dizzy with the eyes closed. She proceeded to the practice of head turning without balance loss while sitting and standing. As both of these goals were accomplished, BP progressed from performing her exercises with head motion and eyes closed while sitting (where there are many somatosensory cues) to quietly standing with a wide

Table 4. Summary of Physical Therapy Treatment

1. Emphasis on enhancing use of information through the somatosensory system and matching that information with visual information
   a. Use of hands and feet against firm surfaces while sitting and standing, looking at a fixation point. Patient concentrates on feeling "still" (not dizzy) with good balance
   b. Lying down, looking at a fixation point on the ceiling and turning the head
   c. Sitting, turning the head using a fixation point
   d. Standing, turning head with a fixation point
2. Establish ability to feel still and not sway with one sensory system absent or reduced
   a. Lying down and progressing to sitting, turning head with eyes closed
   b. Closing the eyes while standing with feet together
   c. Turning head using a fixation point
   d. Standing on foam
   e. Walking while turning head left and right, using fixation point
3. Decreasing sensory cues and continuing to feel "still" and not sway
   a. Standing on one leg, eyes closed
   b. Eye closed, feet together, turn head
   c. Walking with eyes moving left and right (decreases visual input for balance)
   d. Standing on a foam cushion (decreases somatosensory input)

base, then narrowing the base, and finally while walking. To address the problem of imbalance related to vestibular system stimulation (i.e., turning corners or bending over), BP progressed through head turning and bending while sitting, standing and walking until these motions no longer disrupted her balance. By the fourth session (two months later), BP was able to begin the second phase of therapy, during which standing on foam, cushions or pads reduced somatosensory inputs. Finally, BP learned to maintain balance with head movement with and without the eyes open. The final phase of the program involved sensory conflict exercises directed at helping the patient choose the relevant sensation correctly, while ignoring the sensory inputs which were misleading. Sensory conflict exercises involved the use of a moving surface while sitting or standing, and a visually-moving environment while sitting or standing. Movement of the eyes and head during sitting, standing or walking (self motion versus world motion) was used to decrease visual sensitivity. Table 4 summarizes the physical therapy treatment.

Discharge status

Table 1 includes the post-treatment optometric data. The visual acuities, refraction and eye alignment status did not significantly change after rehabilitative treatment. The following showed improvement: nearpoint of convergence, vergences, PRA, stereopsis, cheiroscopic tracings, ocular motilities, and visual/spatial localization. The visual fields normalized.

BP's neurologist noted immediate improvement in balance and movement skills with merely wearing the distance prescription. The small, uncorrected refractive condition had a significant impact on BP's status, as she was extremely dependent on visual cues for balance.

Table 2 shows the post-treatment physical therapy data. BP had normal balance responses, normal gait, was not destabilized with head or eye movements, and reported minimal to no dizziness. Somatosensory input was used normally for balance responses.

Discussion

It is well documented that visual system dysfunctions are frequently found among patients with traumatic brain injury.[9-12, 14-17] When vestibular dysfunction is also present, optimal vision function of the patient is even more important. The patient is often very symptomatic and uncomfortable. In-depth vision and physical therapy evaluations are critical when assessing the injury extent in this population. Particular care is necessary during the optometric evaluation. This often needs to be done slowly and over a period of several sessions, as the patient may become nauseated or dizzy and unable to continue.

The goal of therapy is to improve balance and habituate dizziness and nausea. This is accomplished by enhancing the use of somatosensory inputs and normalizing the visual/ocular functions. Correction of even relatively minor refractive conditions has a major impact with these patients.[18] Rehabilitative VT can improve visual skills and decrease symptomatology.

It is very easy to overload a patient, especially a high-achieving person. Such a patient is motivated to complete a task without paying attention to how he/she is feeling. A patient may become sick for hours or days if overstimulated. Observe the patient's body posture, perspiration, breathing, etc. to detect overstimulation. The patient needs to monitor his/her own level of stimulation throughout therapy.

How dizzy, nauseated or symptomatic should a therapist make a patient? The patient with vestibular dysfunction is learning new strategies and compensations for poor vestibular function. The central nervous system needs an error signal to stimulate this adaptation. In the vestibular patient, dizziness, loss of balance and blurring of vision act as error signals. A patient whose symptoms are not provoked by the therapy program is probably not being stressed enough to force the plastic changes necessary in the central nervous system.[19-21] At the same time, clinicians[22] report that patients whose increased symptoms (dizziness, imbalance, nausea) continue more than three or four days after starting their home therapy do not improve as rapidly as those patients who are back to baseline in this period. It is very easy to overstimulate patients when two or more therapeutic modalities are involved in treatment. In physical therapy, three to five exercises done twice daily (total of ten minutes or less) have been found to be very effective.[23]

Outcomes in these clients are often impressive. For example, in a two-year study of 62 patients with both peripheral and central vestibular dysfunction, 92% reported significantly decreased symptoms and improvement in normal activities of daily living while daily completing ten minutes or less of exercises specifically prescribed for their individual problems.[23]

Why do patients show decreased vestibular symptomatology with rehabilitative VT and PT? The neurophysiological basis for decreased dizziness and improved balance seen in patients is unknown. However, there are several theories or possible explanations for this process. As in BP's case, many patients suffer from abnormalities in vergence, binocular vision and VOR function. Theories presented in the literature to explain the resolution of symptoms by rehabilitative optometric care include:

1. Improvement in function of accommodation and convergence through lenses or prisms because brain-injured patients may lack phoria adaptation [24-25]

2. Improvement in balance between focal and ambient processing systems[26]

3. Improvement in VOR gain with improved refractive status and/or accommodation[27]

4. Integration of erroneous visual information with veridical vestibular and somatosensory information. This results in conflicting sensory information, so that the patient is forced to "choose" a single system for balance

5. Habituation or desensitization may occur to visual surround movement[28]

Physical therapy appears to improve overall function in patients like BP by increasing the use of somatosensory information and decreasing the need for dependency on visual information for balance. Further, the patient is trained to select the most appropriate sensory information in conflicting situations.

Recovery patterns in the brain-injured population often are slower as compared with those patients manifesting peripheral vestibular dysfunction. Symptoms of vestibular dysfunction, including dizziness, nausea, visual hypersensitivity to the environment, and imbalance represent dysfunctions in different pathways in the central nervous system. Patients may improve in all of these areas but at different rates. It is our experience that the dizziness symptoms resolve later, even though a patient resolves the other symptoms earlier. This is most likely because dizziness is caused by flawed integration of the involved sensory systems. Moving in visually-stimulating environments without dizziness or imbalance is often one of the most difficult goals to accomplish. Therefore the individual's visual, somatosensory and vestibular systems must be at higher levels of function to decrease sensory conflict and result in reduced dizziness.

Conclusion

Patients with traumatic brain injury (TBI) frequently exhibit visual system dysfunctions as well as vestibular dysfunction. These patients are often symptomatic and difficult to treat. A combined rehabilitative VT and vestibular PT program can be effective in normalizing clinical findings and reducing symptomatology. More education and referrals between medical physicians and other involved rehabilitation professionals are crucial to improve collaborative treatment for these complex patients.

References

1. Nashner LM. Organization and programming of motor activity during postural control. Prog Brain Res 1979;50:177-84.

2. Nashner L, Shupert CL, Horak F, Black FO. Organization of postural control: an analysis of sensory and mechanical constraints. Prog Brain Res 1989;80:411-8; discussion 395-7.

3. Nolte J. The Human Brain: An Introduction to Its Functional Anatomy. 3rd ed. St. Louis: Mosby Year Book, , 1993:201-17.

4. Herdman S. Vestibular Rehabilitation. 2nd ed. Philadelphia: F.A. Davis, 2000.

5. Shumway-Cook A. Woollacott, M. Abnormal postural control. In: Motor Control: Theory and Practical Applications. Baltimore: Williams & Wilkins, 1995:201.

6. Keshner E. Postural abnormalities in vestibular disorders. In: Herdman S. Vestibular Rehabilitation. 2nd ed. Philadelphia: F.A. Davis, 2000:52-77.

7. Zee D. Vestibular adaptation. In: Herdman S. Vestibular Rehabilitation. 2nd ed. Philadelphia: F.A. Davis, 2000:77-87.

8. Fetter M. Vestibular system disorders. In: Herdman S. Vestibular Rehabilitation. 2nd ed. Philadelphia: F.A. Davis, 2000:91-101.

9. Cohen AH, Rein LD. The effect of head trauma on the visual system: the doctor of optometry as a member of the rehabilitation team. J Am Optom Assoc 1992;63:530-36.

10. Askinoff EB, Falk NS. The differential diagnosis of perceptual deficits in traumatic brain injury patients. J Am Optom Assoc 1992;63:554-58.

11. Tierney DW. Visual dysfunction in closed head injury. J Am Optom Assoc 1988;59:614-22.

12. Hellerstein LF, Freed S, Maples WC. Vision profile of patients with mild brain injury. J Am Optom Assoc 1995;66:634-9.

13. Shumway-Cook A, Olmscheid R. A systems analysis of postural dyscontrol in traumatically brain-injured patients. J Head Trauma Rehabil 1990;5:51-62.

14. Ciuffreda KJ, Suchoff IB, Marrone MA, Ahmann E. Oculomotor rehabilitation in traumatic brain injured patients. J Behav Optom 1996;7:31-8.

15. Langerhorst CT, Safran AB. Progressive shrinkage of the visual field during automated perimetry following traumatic brain injury. Neuro-ophthalmol 1998;20:177-85.

16. Suchoff IB, Kapoor N, Waxman R et al. The occurrence of ocular and visual dysfunctions in an acquired brain injured sample. J Am Optom Assoc 1999;5:301-8.

17. Wainapel SF. Vision rehabilitation: an overlooked subject in physiatric training and practice. Am J Med Rehabil 1995; 74:313-4.

18. Suchoff I, Gianutsos R. Rehabilitative optometric interventions for the adult with acquired brain injury. In: Grabois M, Garrison SJ, Hart KA, Lemkuhl LD, eds. Physical Medicine and Rehabilitation. Malden MA: Blackwall Science, 2000:608-21.

19. Newton RA. Balance abilities in individuals with moderate and severe traumatic brain injury. Brain Injury 1995;9:445-51.

20. Sterm RM, Hu SQ, Vasey MW, Koch KL. Adaptation to vection induced symptoms of motion sickness. Aviat Space Environ Med 1989;60:566-72.

21. Golding JF, Stott JR. Effect of sickness severity on habituation in repeated motion challenges in aircrew referred for airsickness treatment. Aviat Space Envirn Med 1995; 66:625-30.

22. Horak F. Balance Conference, Denver, Co., 1988.

23. Winkler PA. Unpublished data, 1998.

24. North R, Henson DB. The effect of orthoptic treatment upon the vergence adaptation mechanism. Optom Vis Sci 1992 Apr;69(4):294-9.

25. Ogle KN, Matens TG. On the accommodative convergence and proximal convergence. Arch Ophthalmol 1957;57:702.

26. Padula WV. A Behavioral Vision Approach for Persons with Physical Disabilities. Santa Ana, CA: Optometric Extension Program,1988.

27. Ciuffreda K, Tannen B. Eye movement basics for the clinician. St. Louis: Mosby-Yearbook, 1995:112-3.

28. Shepard N, Telian S, Smith-Wetlock M. Habituation and balance retraining therapy; a retrospective review. Neurol Clin 1990;8 (2):459-76.

Index